peaceful places
Chicago

peaceful places
Chicago

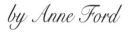

119 Tranquil Sites in

the Windy City and Beyond

by Anne Ford

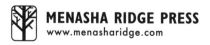

MENASHA RIDGE PRESS
www.menasharidge.com

Copyright © 2011 by Anne Ford
All rights reserved
Published by Menasha Ridge Press
Printed in the United States of America
Distributed by Publishers Group West
First edition, first printing

Cover design by Scott McGrew
Text design by Annie Long
Cartography by Steve Jones
Unless otherwise noted, all interior photographs by Anne Ford
Back cover photographs by Anne Ford
Front cover photograph © David Lyons/Alamy. For a peaceful time to visit the Shedd Aquarium, see page 165.

Library of Congress Cataloging-in-Publication Data

Ford, Anne.
      Peaceful places, Chicago : 110 tranquil sites in the windy city and beyond / Anne Ford.
         p. cm. — (Peaceful places)
      Summary: "The fourth in a new series, each one set in a U.S. metropolis, Peaceful Places:
      Chicago leads the reader on an unexpected path. Author Anne Ford uncovers hidden pockets
      of relaxation throughout the windy city. Her unique guide reveals the surprising gardens, vistas,
      sanctuaries, cafe; respites, and neighborhood strolls that make up Chicago communities from
      downtown to the 'burbs. Readers will discover new destinations, and they will find tips on when
      to visit grand and diminutive locales for a bit of quiet time"—Provided by publisher.
      ISBN-13: 978-0-89732-534-9 (pbk.)
      ISBN-10: 0-89732-534-6 ()
      1. Chicago (Ill.)—Guidebooks. 2. Quietude. I. Title.
      F548.18.F68 2011
      917.73'1104—dc23
                    2011036234

Menasha Ridge Press
P.O. Box 43673
Birmingham, Alabama 35243
menasharidge.com

Disclaimer

Seclusion can be part of the charm of a peaceful place. Likewise, in some locations, the best time to visit is early morning, sunset, or even in the evening, when few other people are around. Therefore, we remind you to maintain awareness and practice caution in all of the destinations described in this book just as you would when venturing to any isolated or unfamiliar location. Please also note that prices, hours, and public transportation routes fluctuate in the course of time and that travel information changes under the impact of many factors that influence the travel industry. We therefore suggest that you write or call ahead for confirmation when making your travel plans. Every effort has been made to ensure the accuracy of information throughout this book, and the contents of this publication are believed to be correct at the time of printing. Nevertheless, the publishers cannot accept responsibility for errors or omissions, for changes in details given in this guide, or for the consequences of any reliance on the information provided by the same. Assessments of sites are based on the author's own experience; therefore, descriptions given in this guide necessarily contain an element of subjective opinion, which may not reflect the publisher's opinion or dictate a reader's own experience on another occasion.

contents

peaceful places alphanumerically

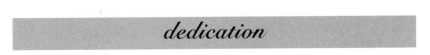

dedication

To David, my peaceful place

acknowledgments

$\mathcal{I}$ am deeply grateful to the many friends who generously suggested their own favorite peaceful places for inclusion here. Among them are Anders Benson, Barbara Bohn, Anthony Burton, Cynthia Dieden, Maureen Jenkins, Penelope Johnson, Andrea Knepper, Stephanie Kuenn, Margaret Littman, Ann Logue, Alison Mankowski, Elizabeth Mankowski, Lynne Marek, Oren Matteson, Michele Means, Liz Morris, Robyn Okrant, Anne Osterman, Jenni Prokopy, Maija Rothenberg, Jorge Sánchez, Anne Stevens, Emily Stone, Beau Surratt, Beth Taylor, Travis Trott, Alison True, John Tryneski, Wendy Vasquez, Lora Walsh, and Constance Wilson. Thanks, too, to my friend and colleague Heather Boerner, whose steadfast companionship from afar made many a writing day easier.

Tremendous gratitude goes to Elaine Glusac for her kindness in connecting me with Menasha Ridge Press, and to editor Susan Haynes for her steady guidance and sure wit.

My wonderful parents deserve all the peacefulness in the world for their unflagging support of me and my writing. And my marvelous stepchildren—Joseph, Rebecca, and Elizabeth—deserve many, many doughnut-related expeditions for their patience with me as I wrote.

This book would not have been possible without the support, enthusiasm, and finely honed navigational abilities of my most amazing husband, David.

introduction

oet Carl Sandburg called Chicago "stormy, husky, brawling . . . alive and strong and coarse and cunning." And he wasn't even talking about driving in the Loop during rush hour. Since the 19th century—when Chicago's population soared from 350 to more than 1 million—the city has borne a reputation as a fast-moving, hard-edged, muscle-bound kind of town. And if you find yourself standing on a downtown street corner beneath the city's famous elevated tracks as a train rumbles overhead and suited-up businesspeople shove past you, it can certainly feel that way.

But there's another side to Chicago, one that doesn't require earplugs and sharp elbows (the better to snag a seat on the El). Busy though it may be, the city positively blossoms with pockets of quiet, if you know where to look. That's what this book is for: to guide you to Chicago's lovely parks, peaceful gardens, placid bookstores, hidden walks, and other places to bask in solitude and serenity.

The destinations represented here consist of places I discovered during my 15-and-counting years as a Chicago-area resident, as well as sites I encountered for the first time in the course of writing this book. It is my hope that you'll not only find new places to explore but also be prompted to visit destinations you've heard of and never quite got around to trying. I can't tell you how many acquaintances of mine have confessed that they've never gone *inside* the beautiful Bahá'í Temple (see page 14), for example, despite frequently driving past it.

And then there's a third category: peaceful spots that are tucked away inside larger, heavily visited attractions. For example, the Smith Museum of Stained Glass Windows (see page 176) at Navy Pier, the Tadao Ando Gallery (see page 190) at The Art Institute, or the Elizabeth Hubert Malott Hall of Jades (see page 45) at the Field Museum. Think of these as your secret getaways for the times you just can't take the crowds.

The good news is that most of the time, finding peace in the city takes only a little effort.

Want to see wild deer? Just take a bus to the Old Edgebrook Historic District (see page 124).

Sit by a 100-year-old ginkgo tree? Then make the easy stroll from Wrigley Field to Warner Park and Gardens (see page 203).

Flip through a first edition of *The Adventures of Sherlock Holmes* in blissful silence? All you have to do is duck into Evanston's Bookman's Alley (see page 22).

Glide on a quiet ice rink more than 1,000 feet above the noisy Magnificent Mile? Head to the 94th floor of downtown's John Hancock Building (see page 170).

Once you start ferreting out moments like these in your everyday life, they seem to be everywhere. And that's when you'll stop thinking of peacefulness as something you can get only on vacation and at great expense.

Anne Ford

Anne Ford
Chicago
September 2011

P.S. This book tells you how to reach destinations by the Chicago Transit Authority (CTA) bus and rail system, Metra commuter rail, and Pace suburban bus service. It generally provides information for public transportation that arrives closest to the destinations. If not available, or where multiple transfers get so complicated that they undermine the tranquil experience, you will see "n/a" (not applicable).

three paths to 119 peaceful places

*I*n *Peaceful Places: Chicago*, author Anne Ford serves up 119 locales for a few hours of quiet time in the greater metro area and farther afield. To make it easy for you to find an entry that suits your mood and desired neighborhood or type of place, we have organized the sites in three different ways:

the path BY CATEGORY

The Peaceful Places by Category guide (see page xvii) organizes the sites into 12 different groups, as listed below. The full text for each destination also includes its category at the top of that individual entry. In many cases it was difficult to classify a place, as it might be a historic site in an outdoor habitat with a scenic vista that feels like a spiritual enclave that is an urban surprise where you can take an enchanting walk! But we tagged each of the sites as seemed most fitting for the focus of the author's description.

Day Trips & Overnights	Outdoor Habitats	Scenic Vistas
Enchanting Walks	Parks & Gardens	Shops & Services
Historic Sites	Quiet Tables	Spiritual Enclaves
Museums & Galleries	Reading Rooms	Urban Surprises

the path BY AREA

The Peaceful Places by Area guide (see page xxii) and maps (see pages xxvi–xxxii) locate sites according to these seven geographic divisions:

Downtown (MAP ONE)

The Loop, Magnificent Mile, Museum Campus, River North, Streeterville, West Loop

North Side (MAP TWO)

Gold Coast, Lake View, Lincoln Park, Lincoln Square, North Park, Old Town, Ravenswood, Rogers Park, Roscoe Village, Uptown, Wrigleyville

West Side (MAP THREE)

East Garfield Park, Edgebrook, Irving Park, River West, Norwood Park, University Village, Wicker Park

South Side (MAP FOUR)

Beverly, Bridgeport, Chinatown, Hyde Park, Near South Side, Pullman, Woodlawn

Northern Suburbs (MAP FIVE)

Evanston, Glencoe, Glenview, Highland Park, Lake Forest, Lincolnwood, Skokie, Waukegan, Wilmette

Western Suburbs (MAP SIX)

Elmhurst, Forest Park, Lisle, Naperville, Oak Park

Farther Afield (MAP SEVEN)

North-central Illinois, Indiana, Wisconsin

the path ALPHANUMERICALLY

Beginning on page 1, each entry unfolds in the main text in alphabetical order and is numbered in sequence. The number travels with that entry throughout the book in the table of contents (see page v), in the Peaceful Places by Category guide (see page xvii), in the Peaceful Places by Area guide (see page xxii), and on the maps (see pages xxvi–xxxii).

PEACEFULNESS RATINGS

Preceding the main text for each profile, listed information notes the entry's category and area. This capsule information also includes the author's rating for the site, on a scale of one to three stars, as follows:

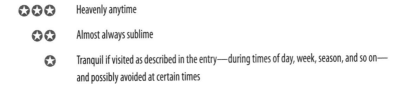

✪✪✪	Heavenly anytime
✪✪	Almost always sublime
✪	Tranquil if visited as described in the entry—during times of day, week, season, and so on— and possibly avoided at certain times

ESSENTIALS

At the end of each entry, you will find the destination's full address, telephone number, website address, cost of entry or a range of prices for menu items or other expenses, hours, and public transportation choices. Note that hours and prices are subject to change, so call to verify before visiting a site.

Regarding public transportation: As the author points out in her introduction, on page xvii, "n/a" (not applicable) denotes destinations not reachable—or not easily accessible—via these services. And as all Chicagoland and other urban dwellers know, public transportation schedules and routes are subject to change. The routes and connections provided are up-to-date at press time, but please check the appropriate websites to be sure you have the latest information for your own journeys.

Throughout Chicago, your leading choices for public transportation are as follows, in alphabetical order, according to the carrier's name:

Chicago Transit Authority (bus and rail)

Metra (commuter rail)

Pace (suburban bus)

For more instructions on the diverse public transportation systems and trip planning in Chicago and the greater Chicago area, visit **rtachicago.com.**

—The Publisher

peaceful places by category

OUTDOOR HABITATS

PARKS & GARDENS

QUIET TABLES

READING ROOMS

SCENIC VISTAS

SHOPS & SERVICES

SPIRITUAL ENCLAVES

URBAN SURPRISES

peaceful places by area

DOWNTOWN (Map One)

NORTH SIDE (Map Two)

NORTHERN SUBURBS (Map Five)

WESTERN SUBURBS (Map Six)

FARTHER AFIELD (Map Seven)

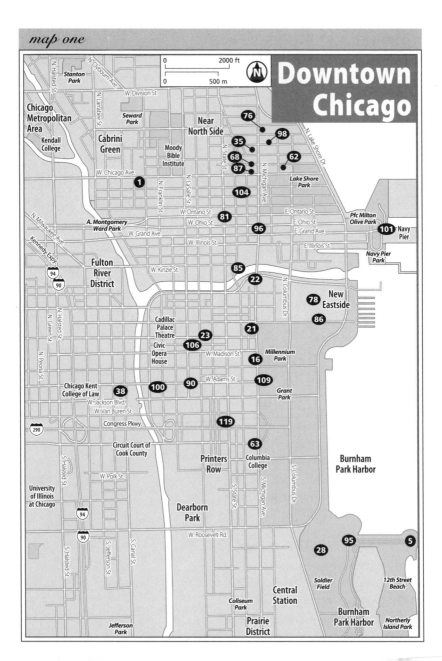

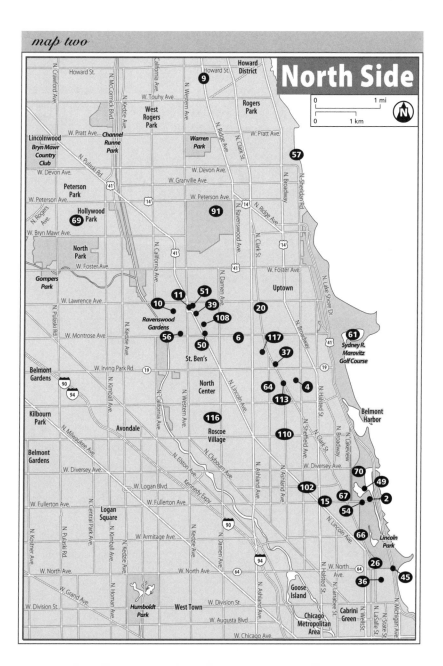

map two

North Side

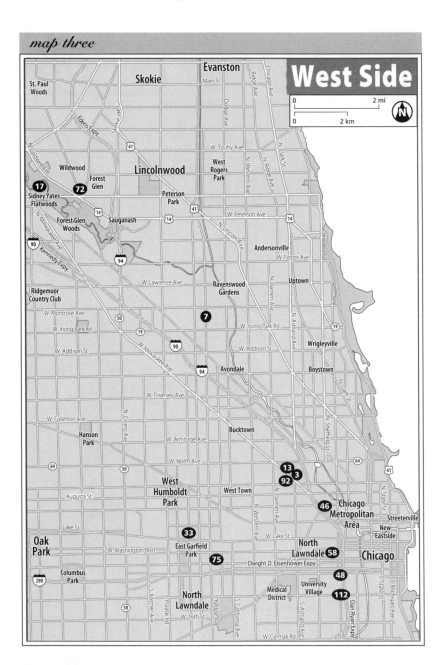

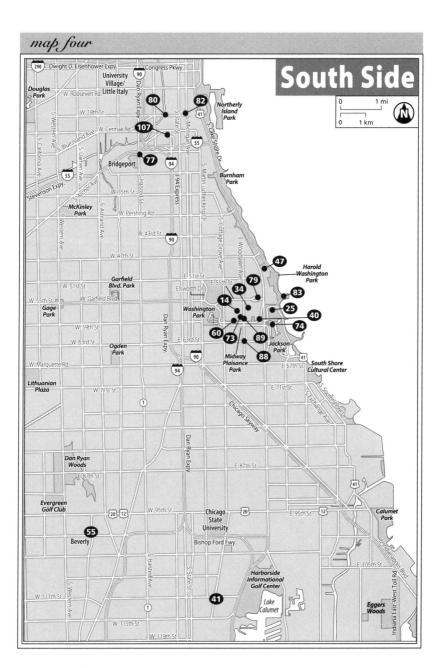

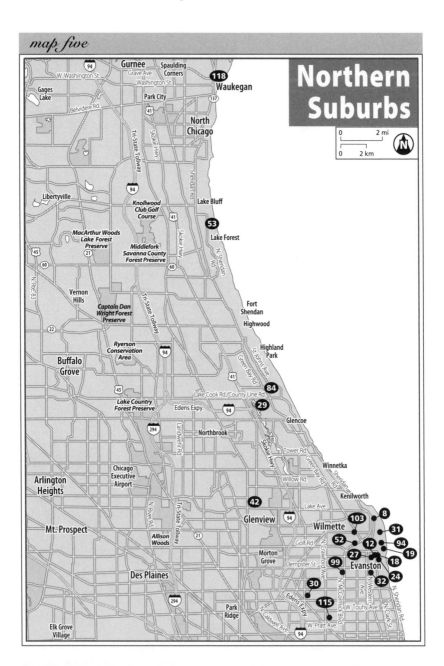

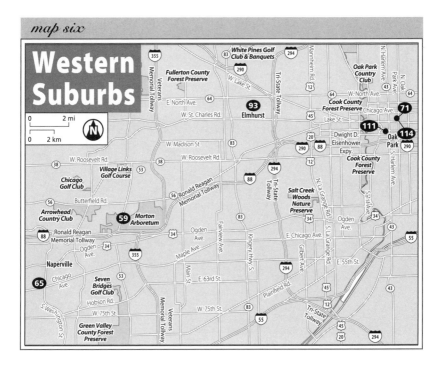

map seven

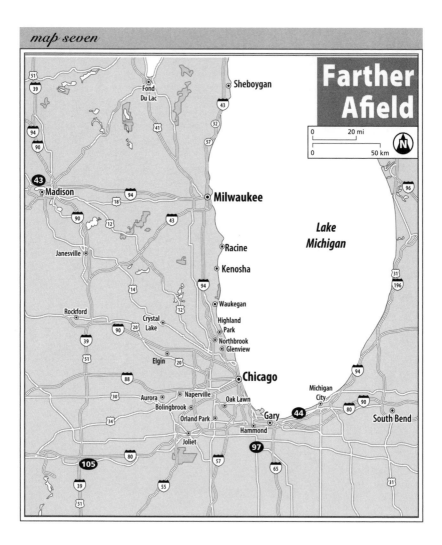

Farther Afield

Sheboygan

Fond
Du Lac

Madison

Milwaukee

*Lake
Michigan*

Racine

Kenosha

Janesville

Waukegan

Rockford

Highland
Park

Crystal
Lake

Northbrook

Glenview

Elgin

Chicago

Michigan
City

Aurora

Naperville

Oak Lawn

Bolingbrook

Orland Park

Gary

South Bend

Hammond

Joliet

0   20 mi

0   50 km

peaceful place 1

ABRAHAM LINCOLN BOOK SHOP

River North, Downtown (MAP ONE)

CATEGORY ⌒ shops & services ✪ ✪

A bookstore, museum, and collectors' delight wrapped into one, this shop—fittingly sited in Illinois, the Land of Lincoln—is famed around the globe as a treasure chest of Lincolniana. It's also a repository of books and historic items related to American presidents in general. Founded in 1938, the shop has resided at its present location for more than 20 years.

Even if you aren't prepared to spend thousands of dollars on, say, a letter hand-written by Andrew Johnson, the staff will happily allow quiet browsing in this subdued, museumlike setting. Items on display vary, but over the years I've seen an impressive array of treasures: an armband that had been worn by a mourner after President Abraham Lincoln's assassination, an engraved invitation to Lincoln's second inaugural ball, and even a scrap of the bloodstained dress that actress Laura Keene is said to have been wearing when she cradled the wounded president's head in her lap after he was shot at Ford's Theatre.

Floor-to-ceiling bookshelves hold both out-of-print and new volumes about American presidential and pre-20th-century military history, and the chairs that dot the store welcome you to sit and read. If you would like to learn more about a given historical topic but are feeling overwhelmed, ask the staff members to get you started. They are quite knowledgeable and always seem happy to help.

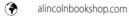 essentials

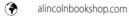 357 West Chicago Avenue, Chicago, IL 60654

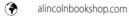 (312) 944-3085

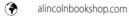 alincolnbookshop.com

$ Free except for purchases

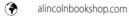 Monday–Wednesday and Friday, 9 a.m.–5 p.m.; Thursday, 9 a.m.–7 p.m.;
Saturday, 10 a.m.–4 p.m.

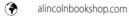 **CTA:** Brown Line, Chicago stop; Bus 66 or 11

peaceful place 2

ALFRED CALDWELL LILY POOL

Lincoln Park, North Side (MAP TWO)

CATEGORY ⌣: parks & gardens ✪ ✪

*I*f this demure lily pool had an advertising jingle, it might be "A Little Piece of Pretty in the Middle of the City." Fortunately for serenity seekers, it keeps a low profile. Duck through the stone entryway on the southwest corner of Fullerton Avenue and Cannon Drive (across the street from the Peggy Notebaert Nature Museum), and you'll feel as if you've tumbled into a secret garden—one filled with wildflowers, birds, wandering stone paths, and of course a tranquil, lily pad–filled pool.

Originally created in 1889, the pool was redesigned in the 1930s by architect Alfred Caldwell, who reputedly cashed in his own life insurance policy to come up with the funds for this mini-oasis. Seven decades later, the many stone terraces surrounding the pool still silently invite passersby to sit and enjoy a quiet moment in the middle of busy Lincoln Park. One drawback, alas, is that while the sights here do an admirable job of shutting out the outside world, the sounds are less successful; that is, traffic is still audible. But concentrate long enough on the ducks tranquilly paddling about the pool or the bright yellow wildflowers scattered alongside, and you'll soon tune it out.

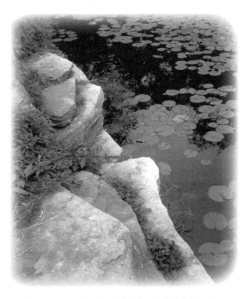

Stone terraces line the Alfred Caldwell Lily Pool.

⌣ essentials

▭ᵗ   Fullerton Avenue and Cannon Drive, Chicago, IL 60614

☏   (312) 742-7726

🌐   chicagoparkdistrict.com (type "lily pool" into the search box)

$ Free

🕓   Daily, April–November, 7 a.m.–7 p.m.

🚌   **CTA:** Red Line, Fullerton stop; Bus 76

peaceful place 3

ALLIANCE BAKERY & CAFÉ

Wicker Park, West Side (MAP THREE)

CATEGORY ⌣ quiet tables ✪ ✪

*W*hat makes this small, arty West Town bakeshop so peaceful? A rather odd architectural setup. The retail area occupies a different storefront than the rest of the café. So you must purchase your meticulously frosted cupcake or adorable French *macaron*, exit onto the sidewalk again, and walk one door down to the completely separate lounge area. This quirk means that customers can hang out, read, work, or go online without the usual coffee shop background clamor of espresso

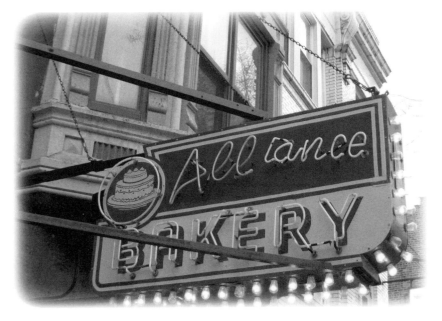

The Alliance Bakery's old-fashioned sign entices visitors inside.

machines, shouted barista conversations, and the like. In the lounge all you'll hear is turning pages, clacking keyboards, very faint background music, and even fainter street noise. It's so quiet here that on a recent visit with a friend, I felt guilty even whispering.

Sit in one of the chairs on the elevated area by the windows, and you'll be able to do some discreet people-watching, courtesy of the gauzy curtains that only partially block the view outside. Alliance guarantees that you'll make the trip back to buy more baked goods by decorating the lounge with photos of their sugary confections.

essentials

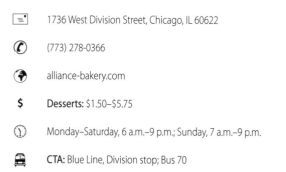

1736 West Division Street, Chicago, IL 60622

(773) 278-0366

alliance-bakery.com

$ **Desserts:** $1.50–$5.75

Monday–Saturday, 6 a.m.–9 p.m.; Sunday, 7 a.m.–9 p.m.

CTA: Blue Line, Division stop; Bus 70

peaceful place 4

ALTA VISTA TERRACE
Wrigleyville, North Side (MAP TWO)
CATEGORY ⌣: enchanting walks ✪ ✪

*O*nly about a 10-minute walk from cacophonous Wrigley Field hides Alta Vista Terrace, one of the most beautiful blocks in the city. Built in 1904, its 40 homes are meant to mimic the row houses of London.

Indeed, if you stumble upon this street during a snowfall, as I recently did, you may fancy yourself transported to a scene from a 19th-century British novel (minus the accents and bowler hats). Though the street is all of one block long, the architectural intricacies of its houses are so captivating that you'll need some time to fully explore

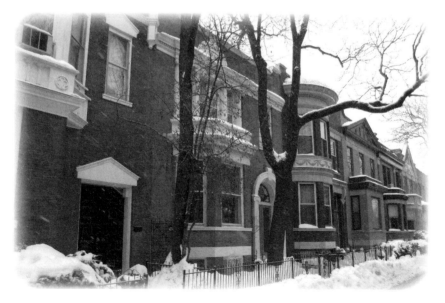

Winter snowscape on Alta Vista Terrace

it. For one thing, the houses sport so many details—bowfront windows, Gothic arches, stained glass pieces, and the like—that it's impossible not to spend time taking them all in. And each house has a mirror-image twin placed diagonally to it, turning a simple stroll down the street into an architectural treasure hunt. Note that parking on Alta Vista Terrace is limited to holders of residential permits, so you'll need to either take public transportation or be willing to park some distance away.

⌣ essentials

🖅	3800 block of North Alta Vista Terrace, Chicago, IL 60613
📞	n/a
🌐	webapps.cityofchicago.org/landmarksweb
$	Free
🕐	Open 24/7
🚌	**CTA:** Red Line, Sheridan stop; Bus 22

AMERICA'S COURTYARD, ADLER PLANETARIUM

Museum Campus, Downtown (MAP ONE)

CATEGORY parks & gardens ✪ ✪

With two floors of fascinating scientific exhibits and a slew of awe-inspiring 3-D documentaries, the Adler rates high on Chicago's list of most valuable cultural institutions. But to enjoy one of the most peaceful experiences it has to offer, you'll have to venture outside its doors. Immediately south of the planetarium, look for the large stone blocks arranged in a spiral. That's *America's Courtyard,* a sculpture that recalls the spiral shape of the Milky Way. (The many different types of stone represented are meant to evoke the diversity of America's peoples, hence the title.)

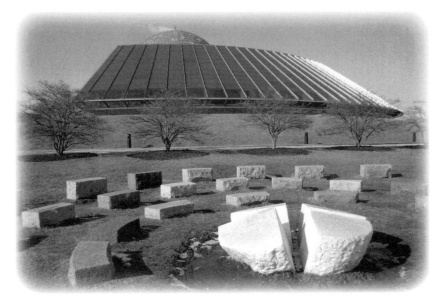

The America's Courtyard *sculpture abuts the Adler Planetarium.*

I like to walk along the curves of the spiral as if in a labyrinth. But you can also take a seat on one of the stones and gaze out at the nearby lake, letting your mind drift free with the water's waves. Or, if you're astronomically inclined, you may enjoy another aspect of the sculpture: the spiral's four avenues leading from the center stones point to the places on the horizon where the sun rises and sets on the June and December solstices each year. As a sign near the sculpture points out, it's possible to track the progress of the seasons this way.

↙ essentials

☐   1300 South Lake Shore Drive, Chicago, IL 60605

✆   (312) 922-7827

🌐   adlerplanetarium.org

$ Free (**planetarium admission:** $10–$27)

🕐   **Planetarium grounds:** Daily, sunrise–sunset.
Planetarium: Monday–Friday, 10 a.m.–4 p.m.; Saturday–Sunday, 10 a.m.–4:30 p.m.
Summer planetarium hours: Daily, 9:30 a.m.–6 p.m.

🚌   **CTA:** Bus 146

peaceful place 6

ARCHITECTURAL ARTIFACTS

Ravenswood, North Side (MAP TWO)

CATEGORY ⌣ shops & services ✪ ✪ ✪

*I*f it weren't for the price tags, you'd mistake this three-floor showroom—which sprawls across two circa 1900 brick buildings—for a museum. A museum of what? Perhaps Americana, antique furniture, architectural pieces, religious artifacts, medical instruments, advertising signs, or stained glass, all of which are well represented among the store's collection of engaging objects. I'm especially fond of the antique glove molds; arranged by the dozen on a display table, they call to mind a crowd of people raising their hands.

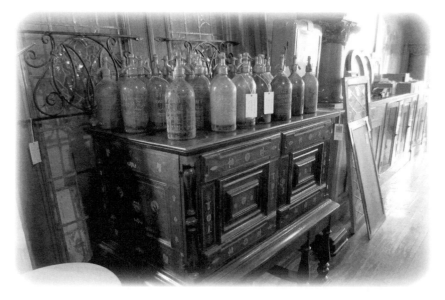

Antique seltzer bottles for sale at Architectural Artifacts

The courteous staff know that many visitors are here to browse, not buy. So feel free to wander as long as you like, whether or not your wallet stretches to a $3,500 1930s-era English phone booth or a $9,500 carnival carousel. If you'd like to pick up a little something without blowing the bank, there are also such small oddities as individual Kodachrome slides or chandelier crystals. The collection here is so vast that you're all but guaranteed a quiet, solitary stroll among the curiosities.

↵ essentials

✉	4325 North Ravenswood Avenue, Chicago, IL 60613
☎	(773) 348-0622
🌐	architecturalartifacts.com
$	Free except for purchases
🕐	Daily, 10 a.m.–5 p.m.
🚌	**CTA:** Brown Line, Montrose stop; Bus 78

peaceful place 7

ARUN'S THAI RESTAURANT
Irving Park, West Side (MAP THREE)
CATEGORY ‿ quiet tables ✪ ✪

*I*n the mood to scarf down a plate of pad thai? This is not the place to go. Arun's serves Thai food, all right, but in a fine-dining setting where patrons enjoy innovative cuisine in a quiet, elegant atmosphere. Come prepared to put yourself in the hands of a master: rather than ordering from a menu, you simply tell your server of any dietary restrictions and—this is important—your tolerance for spice. You'll be served 12 courses: six appetizers, four entrées, and two desserts. (Don't worry; the portions are small enough, and the pauses between courses long enough, that you're left pleasantly full rather than overstuffed.)

The dishes change constantly, but expect flavors and ingredients of curry, lemongrass, coconut, mint, lime, and peanuts. Look, too, for amusing garnishes such as carrot carvings of goldfish and butterflies. The semiprivate dining alcoves add to the pleasure by keeping down the ambient noise. You will find it much easier to appreciate food of this caliber when you are not busy shouting to your companions.

‿ essentials

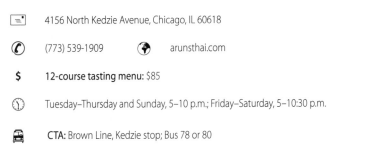

▤ 4156 North Kedzie Avenue, Chicago, IL 60618

✆ (773) 539-1909   ✈ arunsthai.com

$ 12-course tasting menu: $85

🕐 Tuesday–Thursday and Sunday, 5–10 p.m.; Friday–Saturday, 5–10:30 p.m.

🚌 CTA: Brown Line, Kedzie stop; Bus 78 or 80

peaceful place 8

BAHÁ'Í HOUSE OF WORSHIP

Wilmette, Northern Suburbs (MAP FIVE)

CATEGORY ✌ spiritual enclaves ✪ ✪ ✪

*R*ising alongside the broad curves of Sheridan Road like a royal bride, the Bahá'í Temple (as locals call it) represents one of the most stunning sights in the Midwest. Its three-tiered, nine-sided structure is made from crushed quartz and white concrete, poured so skillfully into intricate designs that the dome's sides look like panels of lace draped over marble. Tidy green gardens and sparkling fountains surround the temple.

To reach the domed sanctuary, climb the exterior stairs to the main entrance on the west. Open to all for silent meditation, it's filled with comfortable chairs from which visitors can quietly soak in this elaborate interior. Despite the endless patterns, symbols, and religious sayings (such as, "All the prophets of God proclaim the same truth") that decorate its walls, the space feels light and airy. Look up to see the

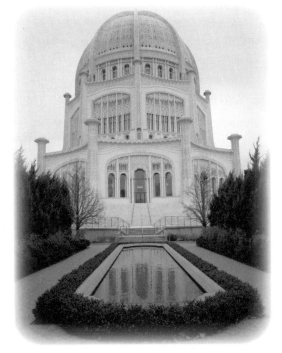

Reflecting pool on the grounds of the Bahá'í House of Worship

Arabic calligraphy that adorns the center of the dome. The wording translates to mean "O Glory of the Most Glorious."

In essence, the Bahá'í faith teaches that God's truth is revealed through all the world's religions. Stroll around the temple's adorned exterior to see that philosophy manifested. You will spot many symbols of Judaism, Buddhism, Christianity, and other faiths. (Don't be alarmed if you see a swastika, which was a religious symbol for centuries before being co-opted by the Nazis.) The site's visitor-information center, in the basement, provides materials for more details on the Bahá'í faith.

✌ essentials

⌷   100 Linden Avenue, Wilmette, IL 60091

☎   (847) 853-2300

⊕   bahai.us

$ Free

🕓   **Sanctuary:** Daily, 6 a.m.–10 p.m.
Visitor center: Daily, 10 a.m.–5 p.m. (open until 8 p.m. during summer).
Devotions: Daily, 9:15 a.m. and 12:30 p.m.

🚌   **CTA:** Purple Line, Linden stop; Bus 201

peaceful place 9

BENEDICTINE SISTERS' ST. SCHOLASTICA MONASTERY LABYRINTH

Rogers Park, North Side (MAP TWO)

CATEGORY ⌣ spiritual enclaves ✪ ✪

*L*ike many of the destinations in this book, the small labyrinth on the grounds of the Benedictine Sisters' St. Scholastica Monastery is easily overlooked unless you know it's there. To find it, take the monastery's service entrance on Ridge Boulevard and look for the white-gravel path past the parking area. A small wooden arch marks the entrance to the labyrinth, which is made of bricks arranged on the ground.

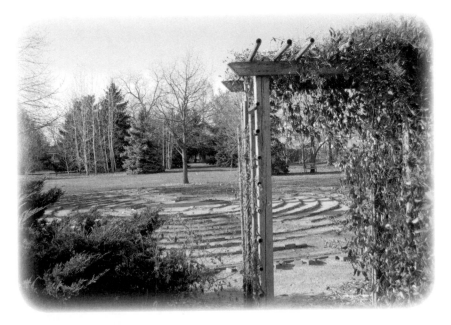

A leafy trellis marks the entrance to the monastery labyrinth.

Once there, walk the labyrinth slowly and contemplatively, following each curve and turning to arrive eventually at the center. Pause as long as you like, and then reverse your steps. It's all intended as a meditative exercise, and indeed, the spiritual analogies abound. For example, the labyrinth's layout makes it seem as if you're closest to the center when you're actually farthest away, and vice versa.

Lying far enough from the road to feel peaceful, the labyrinth is surrounded by trees and benches, so that you can simply sit and contemplate its design if you prefer not to do the walk. Note that the monastery grounds house a school, and that religious groups sometimes visit the labyrinth. Call ahead to make sure that you'll have it to yourself and that, for instance, the track team won't be practicing nearby.

☖ essentials

7430 North Ridge Boulevard, Chicago, IL 60645

(773) 764-2413, ext. 231

osbchicago.org

$ Free

Daily, sunrise–sunset

CTA: Purple Line, Howard stop; Bus 97

peaceful place 10

BLOOM YOGA STUDIO
Lincoln Square, North Side (MAP TWO)
CATEGORY ✌ shops & services ✪ ✪ ✪

*P*racticed serenity seekers know that no matter where they take a yoga class, they're bound to come out feeling more relaxed than when they went in. And, happily, Chicago suffers no shortage of yoga studios. But there's something special about this Lincoln Square yoga center's monthly candlelight yoga classes, generally held on first Fridays in the evening. I recommend seeking them out even if you don't live in the neighborhood.

It's worth the $20 fee for this experience: 90 minutes of *vinyasa* (flowing) poses and stretches in a dimly lit studio accented with the glow of candlelight illumination. Fittingly, rather than the recorded music that accompanies most yoga classes, the candlelight yoga class here relies on live music played by guest musicians on pleasantly exotic instruments such as the didgeridoo and sitar.

Preregistration is recommended for candlelight classes. (However, drop-ins are welcome

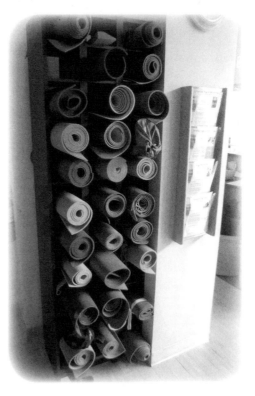

Mats await their yogis at Bloom Yoga Center.

for most other classes; ask at the front desk or see the website for a current schedule.) Also, some yoga experience is recommended, and you can either bring your own mat or rent one for $1.

essentials

✉	4663 North Rockwell Street, Chicago, IL 60625
☎	(773) 463-9642
🌐	bloomyogastudio.com
$	$20
🕐	Generally first Fridays of the month, 8–9:30 p.m.; check schedule on website
🚌	**CTA:** Brown Line, Rockwell stop; Bus 49 or 81

peaceful place 11

THE BOOK CELLAR

Lincoln Square, North Side (MAP TWO)

CATEGORY ⌣ reading rooms ✪

*I*f you love independent bookstores, by all means come here. This cozy shop is the kind of place that features handwritten recommendations posted by staff, library ladders resting against high shelves, and inventory stacked in odd corners. Speaking of odd corners, the best way to maximize the serenity of your experience at The Book Cellar is to skip beyond the front of the store and head for the rear wall. There you'll find two easy chairs—one by the sports section, one by fiction—where you can curl up and

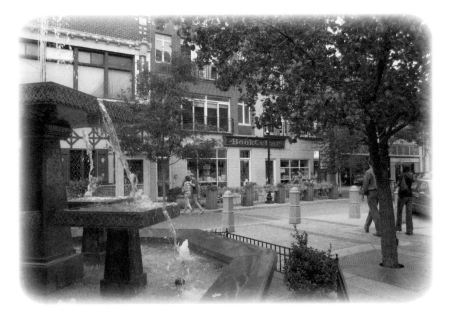

The Book Cellar helps anchor leafy Lincoln Square.

read in peace, with only minimal noise from the store music (though there seem to be no stereo speakers in this area—hurray!).

The store hosts lots of author appearances, book clubs, and other events in the evenings, as well as story times for kids on Friday mornings, so for maximum quietude, come on a weekday afternoon. If you're not averse to a bit of background chatter, the attached café offers a couple of easy chairs, too, as well as sandwiches, pastries, coffee, and even wine by the glass or bottle. Across the street, you'll find another peaceful place mentioned in this book: Kempf Plaza (see page 86).

↵ essentials

4736–38 North Lincoln Avenue, Chicago, IL 60625

(773) 293-2665

bookcellarinc.com

$ Free except for purchases; **café fare:** $4–$7.50

Monday and Wednesday–Saturday, 10 a.m.–10 p.m.;
Sunday and Tuesday, noon–6 p.m.
Summer hours: Monday and Wednesday–Friday, 10 a.m.–10 p.m.;
Saturday, 10 a.m.–11 p.m.; Sunday and Tuesday, 10 a.m.–6 p.m.

CTA: Brown Line, Western stop; Bus 11, 49, or 81

peaceful place 12

BOOKMAN'S ALLEY

Evanston, Northern Suburbs (MAP FIVE)

CATEGORY ⌣ reading rooms ✪ ✪ ✪

*N*ear-silent atmosphere, check. Array of comfortable couches and Oriental rugs, check. Seemingly endless labyrinth of book-stuffed rooms, check. Cheerful octogenarian owner, check. Out-of-the-way back-alley location, check. What this wonderful checklist adds up to is possibly the world's most perfect old-school used bookstore, the kind that was much easier to find before the dawn of Amazon.com.

Owner Roger Carlson, who set up shop in 1979, doesn't seem to care much about raking in the dollars—just about maintaining a haven for serious readers. Some of the tomes in stock are valuable, such as the first edition of *The Adventures of Sherlock Holmes* I saw on a recent visit. Others fall into the $8–$20 range, and still others sit on

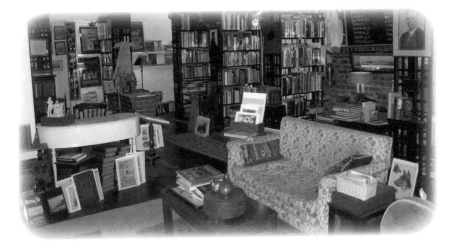

The living room–like atmosphere at Bookman's Alley

the shelves marked "cheap," "cheaper," or "cheapest," where they sell for $1–$3 or so. Reading the shelf labels here is nearly as entertaining as browsing the books themselves. My favorite is "The Joy of Sets," which adorns a shelf holding several matching volumes. To find the shop, look for the alley that links Sherman and Benson avenues just north of Church Street.

essentials

✉	1712 Sherman Avenue (rear), Evanston, IL 60201
☎	(847) 869-6999
🌐	n/a
$	Books begin at $1
🕐	Tuesday–Friday and Sunday, noon–6 p.m.; Saturday, 10:30 a.m.–6 p.m.
🚌	**CTA:** Purple Line, Davis stop; Bus 201

peaceful place 13

THE BORING STORE

Wicker Park, West Side (MAP THREE)

category ⌣ shops & services ✪ ✪

*T*o understand the joke behind this small shop's name, as well as its motto ("The Least Intriguing Retail Outlet in the Midwest"), you need to know that it's more than a store. It's actually the retail side of 826CHI, the Chicago branch of a nationwide organization that provides free writing classes and homework help to students from kindergarten through high school. Classes and tutoring take place in the writing center that adjoins the store, which sells novelty "spy" supplies such as fake mustaches and disappearing ink. It's called The Boring Store so that no one will suspect your secret-agent mission—get it?

The real secret is that because most of the student services are provided after school, the store remains pretty quiet for much of the day. You can quietly browse the entertaining goods, which include rearview sunglasses, trench coats, and tiny mustaches that you apply to the side of your finger (just hold your finger beneath your nose, and voilà—instant disguise). The shop also sells books of the students' creative writing, including the hilarious *A Sunday Afternoon Hot-Dog Meal*, a travel guide to Chicago written entirely by kids.

⌣ essentials

🖃	1331 North Milwaukee Avenue, Chicago, IL 60622
ℰ	(773) 772-8108 ⟲ notasecretagentstore.com
$	Free except for purchases; **items:** $3–$45
🕐	Monday–Thursday, noon–6 p.m.; Friday–Sunday, 11 a.m.–5 p.m.
🚌	CTA: Blue Line, Division stop; Bus 56

peaceful place 14

BOTANY POND
Hyde Park, South Side (MAP FOUR)
category ⌣ outdoor habitats ✪ ✪

*W*hen I was in graduate school at the University of Chicago, I passed this pond near the main quadrangles almost every day. But not until a mama duck and her brood of tiny, fluffy quackers took up residence one spring did I stop and realize how rich with life it really is. (I wasn't the only gawker, either—those little ducklings drew quite a nature-loving crowd.)

Fish, red-eared slider turtles, and gauzy-winged dragonflies make frequent appearances, while redbud trees and other vegetation give it all a lush, fertile feel. From the little bridge over the pond (a very popular site for romantic photographs), you can look down to watch plump goldfish dart beneath the pale, fragrant water lilies. Nearby benches make it possible to spend a quiet hour or more enjoying the scenery, reading, or picnicking. If you've forgotten your lunch, the close-by Reynolds Club houses several eateries. For that matter, if your trip to Botany Pond gets rained out, the club's large, quiet first-floor lounge is a peaceful oasis in its own right (albeit one without ducklings or dragonflies).

⌣ essentials

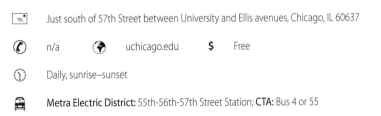

⌨ Just south of 57th Street between University and Ellis avenues, Chicago, IL 60637

🕐 n/a   🌏 uchicago.edu $ Free

🕐 Daily, sunrise–sunset

🚌 **Metra Electric District:** 55th-56th-57th Street Station; **CTA:** Bus 4 or 55

peaceful place 15

BOURGEOIS PIG CAFÉ
Lincoln Park, North Side (MAP TWO)
category ⌣ quiet tables ✪ ✪

*B*y unspoken agreement, the small south-facing room on the top floor of this old-house-turned-coffee-shop is the quiet zone. Other areas, including the outdoor patio, are reserved for chattering college students from neighboring DePaul University. Order some food at the counter downstairs, if you like; then climb the foot-worn staircase, take a left through the French doors, and settle in at one of the wooden tables. Better still, head for a comfy curved-back couch. If you've forgotten reading material, help yourself to one of the antique tomes conveniently littered about (recently spotted: *Mental Health through Will-Training*). Perhaps rest your feet with a sigh on the steamer trunk that serves as a coffee table.

The vast menu here at the Pig, as it is known, includes dozens of hearty sandwiches named after books: Old Man and the Sea (made with tuna salad flavored with fresh dill) is one tasty example. Or try The

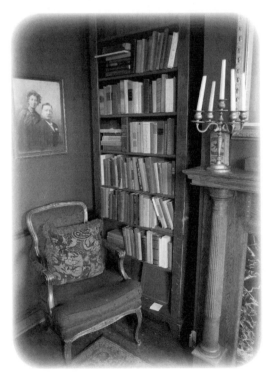

A quiet corner at the Bourgeois Pig

Secret Garden (avocado, tomato, cucumber, and sprouts on multigrain). By way of simpler pleasures, there's a vast loose-leaf tea selection, plus a motley assortment of baked goods. In my opinion, the Pig's only downside is its unreliable Internet service (which is free with a purchase), but even that has a silver lining: fewer laptop luggers to hog the tables.

✌ essentials

738 West Fullerton Parkway, Chicago, IL 60614

(773) 883-5282

bpigcafe.com

Sandwiches: $7.45–$11.95

Monday–Saturday, 7 a.m.–10 p.m.; Sunday, 8 a.m.–10 p.m.

CTA: Red Line, Fullerton stop; Bus 74

peaceful place 16

BP BRIDGE AND LURIE GARDEN, MILLENNIUM PARK

The Loop, Downtown (MAP ONE)

category ꙳ parks & gardens ✪

*E*ver since Millennium Park opened in 2004, Chicagoans have largely come to identify it with its most prominent features: the slick, kidney-shaped *Cloud Gate* sculpture (also known as The Bean) by British artist Anish Kapoor; the reflecting pool and digital displays of the Crown Fountain; and the free ice rink that draws thousands of skaters each winter. However, the park offers less conspicuous but equally pleasant features too—and their lower profiles mean fewer crowds.

To find these attractions, make your way to the park's southeast section and look for the entrance to the BP Bridge. This shiny, serpentine footbridge, which leads to Daley

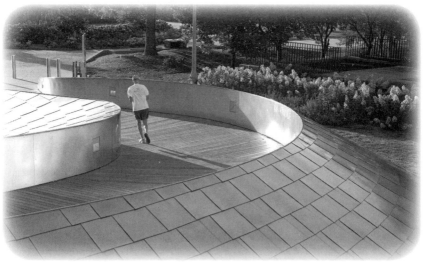

A lone jogger traverses the BP Bridge.

Bicentennial Plaza, acts as a barrier against traffic noise. Something about its sinuous curves makes walking across it a mildly meditative experience. After you return to the bridge's entry point, look for the narrow canal just to the south and follow it to the Lurie Garden. Its riotous wildflowers and prairie grasses yield an unexpectedly wild effect, especially in contrast to the urban landscape outside the park. Depending on the time of year, look for crocuses, daylilies, bluebells, meadow sage, and more.

✓ essentials

Michigan Avenue and Monroe Street, Chicago, IL 60603
Welcome Center: 201 East Randolph Street, Chicago, IL 60601

(312) 742-1168

millenniumpark.org

$ Free

Daily, 6 a.m.–11 p.m.

Metra Electric District: Millennium Station; **CTA:** Red Line, Monroe stop; Bus 151

peaceful place 17

CALDWELL WOODS

Norwood Park, West Side (MAP THREE)

category ↶ outdoor habitats ✪ ✪

*P*art of the Cook County Forest Preserve, Caldwell Woods is perhaps best known as the starting point of the North Branch Bike Trail. The two-lane paved trail leads about 14 miles north through several other areas of the preserve. It winds through trees and along the Chicago River all the way to the Chicago Botanic Garden—a satisfying biking or in-line-skating outing for a spring, summer, or fall day. (Keep an eye out for deer as you zip by; they dwell in the preserve in considerable numbers.)

If you'd like to stay a little more local, Caldwell Woods offers wide-open swaths of land perfect for tossing a Frisbee around with a friend or having a picnic, as well as great sledding slopes on snowy days. From the parking area just off Devon Avenue, you'll walk down a set of cement stairs to reach the woods, meaning that once you're down there, traffic is all but invisible—making a visit here feel like an escape from the city. (I do recommend bringing a companion on any excursion to the woods, as they can feel highly isolated.)

↶ essentials

▤	6200 West Devon Avenue, Chicago, IL 60645
☎	(800) 870-3666
🌐	fpdcc.com
$	Free
🕐	Daily, sunrise–sunset
🚍	**Metra Union Pacific:** Northwest Line, Norwood Park Station; **CTA:** Bus 68

peaceful place 18

CELTIC KNOT PUBLIC HOUSE

Evanston, Northern Suburbs (MAP FIVE)

category ✄ quiet tables ✪ ✪

*A*n Irish pub may not sound like your idea of a quiet retreat, but it all depends on your timing. While a Friday or Saturday evening at this cozy Evanston spot is likely to be both loud and lively, there's an easy way to experience the charm of the Celtic Knot under quieter circumstances: afternoon tea. The pub lies only a few minutes' walk away from another peaceful Evanston destination, the Close Knit yarn shop (see page 40). Why not combine the two for a satisfying afternoon out?

Available on Wednesday and Saturday afternoons, Moira's Afternoon Tea, as it's billed, serves up plate upon plate of petite sandwiches, scones, cream puffs, pastries, and more—all in a peaceful, low-key atmosphere. And the service underscores your

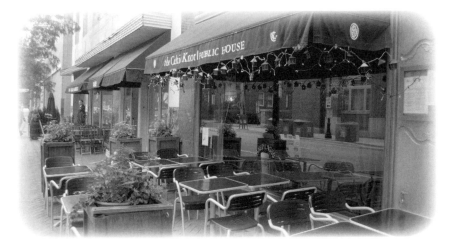

Sidewalk seating at the Celtic Knot

experience, as the attentive staff frequently bustle out of the kitchen to make sure that your brew stays hot. Unlike afternoon tea at the large downtown Chicago hotels, which can run $35 and up per person, here it's no pricier than a decent lunch. (Your meal will consist of three sandwiches, one scone with Kerry Gold butter, three pastries, and unlimited tea.) There's a half-price kids' option too. In warm weather, outdoor seating is available at sidewalk tables, though be warned that you'll lose a little ambience (as the pub sits on a busy street).

↙ essentials

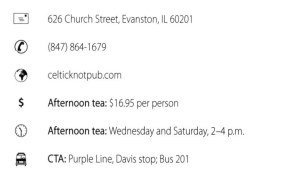

▤   626 Church Street, Evanston, IL 60201

☏   (847) 864-1679

🌐   celticknotpub.com

$ **Afternoon tea:** $16.95 per person

🕐   **Afternoon tea:** Wednesday and Saturday, 2–4 p.m.

🚌   **CTA:** Purple Line, Davis stop; Bus 201

peaceful place 19

CHARLES DEERING LIBRARY
Evanston, Northern Suburbs (MAP FIVE)
category ∿ reading rooms ✪ ✪ ✪

*W*hen you're in desperate need of an absolutely silent retreat, try Deering. Once Northwestern's sole library, the beautiful Gothic building now holds the university's music, art, map, and special collections, as well as its institutional archives. Don't make the mistake of trying to access this fortress of learning through its own

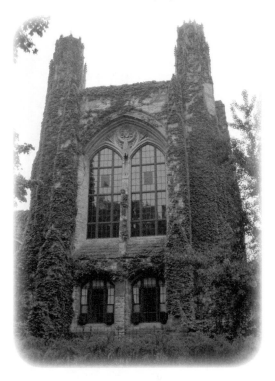

The Charles Deering Library's ivy-covered edifice

doors: visitors must enter the main, modern library just adjacent to it. Walk to the end of a rather nondescript hallway, where a sign helpfully points out HIDDEN STAIRS TO PRETTY PART OF DEERING, that is, the second and third floors. They are worth the climb.

On both floors you'll find lovely, silent reading rooms filled with long wooden tables and flanked by enormous arched windows. In the Art Collection room, take time to stroll the perimeter and look at the painted window medallions, which feature a hodgepodge of images from the Holy Grail to a genie in a bottle. Look, too, for the antique wooden printing press that graces the third-floor lobby. Or just settle down with a book at one of the tables and bask in the utter quiet. Note that the library's hours fluctuate during summer and holiday periods, and that the hours for the general public (see below) differ from the hours for students.

↩ essentials

⊟	1970 Campus Drive, Evanston, IL 60208
☎	(847) 491-7658
🌐	library.northwestern.edu
$	Free
🕐	**General public hours:** Monday–Friday, 8:30 a.m.–5 p.m.; Saturday, 8:30 a.m.–noon
🚇	**CTA:** Purple Line, Foster stop; Bus 201

peaceful place 20

CH'AVA CAFÉ
Uptown, North Side (MAP TWO)
category ↙ quiet tables ✪ ✪

*B*ecause I'm an urban-dwelling writer, coffee shops are my native habitat—
and I've been to so many of them in and around Chicago that I can attest
with certainty to Ch'ava's distinctiveness. Many coffee shops (and I'm not knocking
them) seem to subscribe to the dark-and-cozy theory of interior decorating. In contrast,
Ch'ava's futuristic decor and chill white walls give it a vibe best described as where the
Jetsons go to get away from it all.

At the same time, playful details such as lime-green lamps keep it from feeling sterile
or bland. Perhaps most miraculously, the lively setting doesn't result in an overly chatty
atmosphere. Even on a Sunday morning, I'm able to relax here without being driven nuts
by background babble. Another peace-producing feature is the café's adjacent parking
lot, which allows you to spend an afternoon here without having to run out and feed the
meter every 2 hours. The food is top-notch, too, with sophisticated fare such as braised
short rib sandwiches, oyster mushroom sandwiches, and spicy cold tomato soup.

↙ essentials

🖃	4656 North Clark Street, Chicago, IL 60640
✆	(773) 942-6763
🌐	chavacafe.com
$	**Salads and sandwiches:** $4.99–$10.99
🕐	Monday–Friday, 7 a.m.–10 p.m.; Saturday–Sunday, 8 a.m.–10 p.m.
🚌	**CTA:** Red Line, Lawrence stop; Bus 22

peaceful place 21

CHICAGO PUBLISHERS GALLERY & CAFÉ, CHICAGO CULTURAL CENTER

The Loop, Downtown (MAP ONE)

category ↙ reading rooms ⭐

$\mathscr{M}$any Chicagoans, especially those who work in the Loop, think of the Cultural Center as a place to hear an occasional free lunchtime concert. But the center offers other opportunities to relax and take a load off too. One such choice is the Publishers Gallery, a large reading room in which all the available books have been published by a press in the Chicago area. While borrowing or buying books isn't allowed, patrons are welcome to sit and peruse as long as they like. And there are plenty of selections, from the famous *Chicago Manual of Style* to *The Night Bookmobile,* a graphic novel by Audrey Niffenegger, the Chicago-based author of *The Time Traveler's Wife.* A kids' corner keeps young ones happy. The enormous SILENCE sign on the wall helps keep down the low-level chatter. If you need to escape even that, head upstairs to take in one of the rotating special cultural exhibits or to have a peek at the enormous Tiffany stained glass dome, said to be the largest in the world.

↙ essentials

📧   78 East Washington Street, Chicago, IL 60602   📞   (312) 744-6630

🌐   chicagoculturalcenter.org (click on "Other Things to Do," and look for Publishers Gallery in the list)

$ Free

🕐   Monday–Thursday, 8 a.m.–7 p.m.; Friday, 8 a.m.–6 p.m.; Saturday, 9 a.m.–6 p.m.; Sunday, 10 a.m.–6 p.m.

🚌   **CTA:** Brown Line, Randolph/Wabash stop; Blue Line, Washington stop; Bus 151

peaceful place 22

THE CHICAGO RIVERWALK

Downtown (MAP ONE)

category ⌇ enchanting walks ✪ ✪

*W*hen I visit Chicago's Riverwalk—the paved walkway that runs beneath Michigan Avenue and Lake Shore Drive and extends from State Street to the lake—I waver between disbelief that more people don't use it and gratitude that they don't. But if you're familiar with San Antonio's famous Riverwalk, don't come here anticipating a similarly built-up, commercial atmosphere. Aside from a few cafés,

photographed by Kate Joyce/Hedrich Blessing Photographers;
courtesy of Ross Barney Architects

The Michigan Avenue Bridge, as seen from the Chicago Riverwalk

boat-tour operators, and bike-rental outfits, Chicago's version is a quiet, near-pristine place, highly amenable to a peaceful stroll.

After descending one of the staircases at the Michigan Avenue Bridge and beginning to walk east toward the lake, you'll spot several opportunities for relaxation: a group of chairs invites you to sit and gaze at the water, Cyrano's café sells wine by the glass, another place rents out bicycles built for two (or even four), and an outfit called the Spa Stop offers back and foot rubs. Or you can just keep strolling to the Riverwalk's end, where you can sit on a bench, watch sailboats in the harbor, and become mesmerized by the Ferris wheel at nearby Navy Pier.

⌣ essentials

📧   Chicago River along Wacker Drive between State Street and Lake Michigan, Chicago, IL 60601

📞   n/a

🌐   cityofchicago.org

$ Free

🕐   Daily, 6 a.m.–11 p.m.

🚌   **CTA:** Red Line, Lake stop; Bus 151

peaceful place 23

THE CHICAGO TEMPLE

The Loop, Downtown (MAP ONE)

category ⌁ spiritual enclaves ✪ ✪ ✪

*T*hough the building's name may suggest an exotic air, this lofty site in the heart of the Loop rather matter-of-factly houses the First United Methodist Church. The room for which the temple is most famous—the Sky Chapel—is, at 400 feet above street level, said to be the highest place of worship in the world. Unfortunately, that enticement is open to the public only for worship services and free tours at 2 p.m. Monday–Saturday and after each Sunday service. But to the casual visitor simply looking for a spot to rest, read, or meditate, that's no matter, as the lovely first-floor main sanctuary allows all three—resting, reading, and meditating.

To reach this haven, enter on the Washington Street side of the Chicago Temple, and keep walking straight until you see the large QUIET, PLEASE sign that indicates the sanctuary entrance. Once you're inside, the heavy doors ensure that none of the activity in the entryway vicinity is audible. Dark wooden pews, subdued stained glass windows, and a simple altar flanked by candles create an environment of beautiful minimalism that inspires contemplation.

⌁ essentials

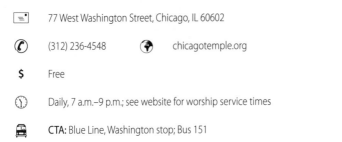

⌨ 77 West Washington Street, Chicago, IL 60602

☏ (312) 236-4548   🌐 chicagotemple.org

$ Free

🕐 Daily, 7 a.m.–9 p.m.; see website for worship service times

🚌 **CTA:** Blue Line, Washington stop; Bus 151

peaceful place 24

CLOSE KNIT

Evanston, Northern Suburbs (MAP FIVE)

category ↙ shops & services ✪ ✪

A good knitting shop isn't just a place to buy yarn and needles. It's a jewel box filled with tiny discoveries, from hand-dyed merino wool to one-of-a-kind patterns, and it's staffed by patient, helpful people. That description fits Close Knit like a handmade glove. Floor-to-ceiling shelves are laden with yarns of myriad weights and colors, with the more expensive specialty fibers heaped in baskets in the middle.

The sweet owner or one of her staffers will bend over backwards to help knitters find the perfect yarn or pattern. Even if you don't knit, you may decide to take it up after seeing the peaceful scene of knitters sitting around the store's table, working on their crafts and chatting in quiet companionship. If you do decide to try your hand at it, ask about the in-store classes aimed at all skill levels. If you don't knit and don't want to start, it's still worth stepping into this quiet, colorful haven, if only to enjoy the atmosphere and browse through the many hand-knit items for sale.

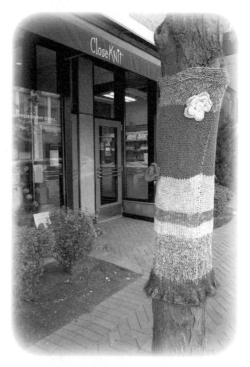

Even the trees wear sweaters near yarn shop Close Knit.

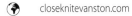 essentials

⊡   531 Davis Street, Evanston, IL 60202

✆   (847) 328-6760

🌐   closeknitevanston.com

$ Free except for purchases

🕐   Monday–Tuesday, 11 a.m.–6 p.m.; Wednesday and Friday, 11 a.m.–5 p.m.;
      Thursday, 11 a.m.–7 p.m.; Saturday, 11 a.m.–4:30 p.m.;
      Sunday, noon–4 p.m. (closed on Sunday during summer)

🚌   **CTA:** Purple Line, Davis stop; Bus 201

peaceful place 25

COLLEEN MOORE'S FAIRY CASTLE, MUSEUM OF SCIENCE AND INDUSTRY

Hyde Park, South Side (MAP FOUR)

category ↙ museums & galleries ✪

*S*cience is fun, but it's not quiet—at least, not at this überpopular Chicago institution. There's just so much for kids to do and see and smell and touch and jump on here that the noise level seldom falls below hectic. But at least one lovely pocket of calm does exist: the room dedicated to Colleen Moore's Fairy Castle. The most fanciful and expensive dollhouse you're ever likely to see, this pet project of silent film star Colleen Moore sits in a darkened enclave on the museum's lower level. The occasional group of noisy visitors does come in but rarely lingers; there's too much detail here to capture the attention of the impatient ones. The castle holds more than 2,000 miniatures, from the copper stove in the kitchen (meant to represent the one from "Hansel and Gretel") to Cinderella's wee glass slippers. My favorite room: the jewel-jammed cave of Ali Baba, reachable to the castle's imaginary inhabitants only by trapdoor. Audio receivers on each side of the display allow you to hear a recorded explanation of every room's tiny delights.

↙ essentials

📧   57th Street and Lake Shore Drive, Chicago, IL 60637

📞   (773) 684-1414   🌐   msichicago.org

$ Adults and children age 12 and older: $13–$27; **seniors age 65 and older:** $12–$26; **children ages 3–11:** $9–$18

🕐   Daily, 9:30 a.m.–4 p.m. (extended hours on select dates; see website for details)

🚌   **Metra Electric District:** 55th-56th-57th Street Station; **CTA:** Bus 2, 6, 10, or 55

peaceful place 26

DIORAMA HALL, CHICAGO HISTORY MUSEUM
Old Town, North Side (MAP TWO)
category ↙ museums & galleries ✪ ✪

*T*he Chicago History Museum has done a great job of bringing the past to life with hands-on experiences. Here you can make your own giant Chicago-style hot dog, sit in a seat from the old Comiskey Park, board a vintage Chicago elevated train car (or El car), listen to blues music that originated here, and more.

But if it's peace and quiet you're after, then head directly to the Diorama Hall on the first floor, straight back and to the left of the museum entrance. The hall contains seven stunning dioramas, each depicting a different period of Chicago's rich history. The scenes offer incredible detail: you can spot a gondolier on a lagoon in the 1893 World's Columbian Exposition, see dancers twirling inside the Sauganash Tavern (Chicago's first hotel), and— thanks to some skillful lighting—watch realistic flames of the Great Chicago Fire sweep over the city. Not only does the dim lighting in the hall make it easier to see the glassed-off dioramas, but it also lends a hushed, contemplative mood. Then, too, the Diorama Hall's relative seclusion from the rest of the museum means that unless you stumble upon a visiting school group, or they stumble upon you, the noise level here is minimal.

↙ essentials

⌨ 1601 North Clark Street, Chicago, IL 60614

☎ (312) 642-4600   ✈ chicagohistory.org

$ Adults: $14; seniors age 65 and older and students ages 13–22 with ID: $12; children age 12 and younger and museum members: free

☽ Monday–Saturday, 9:30 a.m.–4:30 p.m.; Sunday, noon–5 p.m.

🚌 CTA: Red Line, Clark/Division stop; Bus 22 or 36

peaceful place 27

DREAM ABOUT TEA

Evanston, Northern Suburbs (MAP FIVE)

category ༈ quiet tables ✪ ✪

*G*olden Silk. Milk Fragrance. Silver Needle. Even before you take a single sip, the names of the teas in this store let you know that you're not in Starbucks anymore, Toto. What the small, haphazardly decorated shop lacks in decor and food (it sells only a few pastries and such), it more than makes up for with its broad and exotic tea menu, as well as with its peaceful atmosphere. Even the hearty Chinese black teas are designed to make you slow down; their unfiltered leaves float in your cup, forcing you to drink unhurriedly and deliberately. If you prefer a cup of Earl Grey, never fear—English teas are on offer too. Feel free to ask the counter workers for recommendations; they are intimately familiar with their wares and happy to steer you in your chosen direction (strong? sweet? minty?).

Take a seat at one of the several small tables, or call ahead to reserve the more comfortable couch. Or wander around the store with your teacup, browsing through the imported tea paraphernalia for sale, such as clay teapots or bamboo strainers from China.

༈ essentials

🖃	1011 Davis Street, Evanston, IL 60201
✆	(847) 864-7464
🌐	dreamabouttea.com
$	**Tea:** $2.75–$6.75
🕐	Tuesday–Saturday, 11 a.m.–7 p.m.; Sunday, noon–6 p.m.
🚍	**CTA:** Purple Line, Davis stop; Bus 201

peaceful place 28

ELIZABETH HUBERT MALOTT HALL OF JADES, FIELD MUSEUM

Museum Campus, Downtown (MAP ONE)

category ⌣ museums & galleries ✪

*G*et as far as you can from the dinosaurs—that's my advice to anyone looking for a quiet spot of contemplation inside the enormous, fascinating Field Museum. Visitors of all ages and excitability quotients seem inexorably drawn to the *Tyrannosaurus rex* skeleton known as Sue, along with the other dinosaur fossils on display here.

So when you seek a breather from the crowds, head to the south end of the top floor, well away from Sue and her ilk (as fascinating as they are), and ensconce yourself in the Hall of Jades. Really a medium-size room made atmospheric by muted lighting, the hall

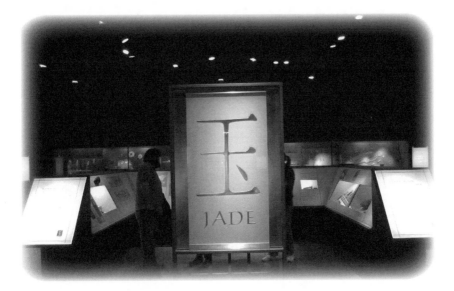

Dimly lit treasures in the Hall of Jades

showcases hundreds of intriguing jade artifacts, some dating back to 3300 BC. Here you'll learn how white jade was reserved for emperors, how high-ranking officials during the Han period were buried in special suits made from thousands of small jade plates, and why this extremely durable stone symbolized longevity to the ancient Chinese. Visitors can even touch a jade boulder weighing 2,490 pounds. Best of all, the atmosphere in this room is pleasantly hushed, giving new meaning to the term *stone silence.*

Afterward, if you'd like to prolong the relative quiet a little longer, head just across the way to the Grainger Hall of Gems. There, you can have a similarly undisturbed experience.

⌣ essentials

    ▣   1400 South Lake Shore Drive, Chicago, IL 60605

    ✆   (312) 922-9410

    🌍   fieldmuseum.org

    $ Adults: $15–$29; seniors age 65 and older and students with ID: $12–$24; children ages 3–11: $10–$20

    🕐   Daily, 9 a.m.–5 p.m.

    🚌   **CTA:** Bus 146

ELIZABETH HUBERT MALOTT JAPANESE GARDEN, CHICAGO BOTANIC GARDEN

Glencoe, Northern Suburbs (MAP FIVE)

category ↵ enchanting walks ✪ ✪

The English Walled Garden is pristine; the Model Railroad Garden is intricate; the Aquatic Garden, with its water lilies and ducks, is just plain lovely. But, hands down, for the most serene experience within the Chicago Botanic Garden, walk through the Japanese Garden, admiring its curving paths, precisely trimmed pine trees, and mirrorlike lake as you go. The garden is laid out so that with each turn in the path, a new vista opens up to you, making this walk as engaging as it is tranquil. A zigzag bridge forces you to slow your steps and take in the view of the lake, rather than just hurrying across. Alas, no bridge allows you to cross to Horaijima, termed the lake's "island of everlasting happiness"; as lovely as it is, you must view it from afar.

I particularly enjoy the site's dry garden—an arrangement

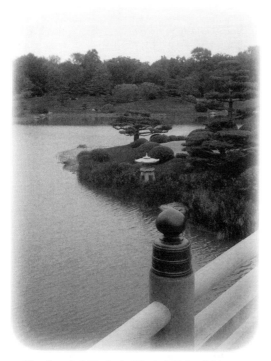

View from the bridge in the Elizabeth Hubert Malott Japanese Garden

of rocks and carefully raked gravel that has a strange power to soothe the mind of onlookers. Many visitors like the Japanese Garden best in winter, when snow blankets the landscape and makes everything appear even more still and serene.

⌣ essentials

✉	1000 Lake Cook Road, Glencoe, IL 60022
☎	(847) 835-5440
🌐	chicagobotanic.org
$	Free admission; $20 per car parking fee
🕐	Daily, 8 a.m.–sunset. **Summer hours:** Daily, 7 a.m.–9 p.m.
🚌	**Metra Union Pacific:** North Line, Braeside Station; **Pace:** Bus 213

peaceful place 30

EMILY OAKS NATURE CENTER

Skokie, Northern Suburbs (MAP FIVE)

category ↙ outdoor habitats ✪ ✪

his nature center and restored savanna styles itself as "your next-door nature place," and with good reason. It sits in an unassuming residential neighborhood and, at just 13 acres, is small enough that a visit here doesn't require a major chunk of time (or any gear besides decent walking shoes). The main draw: a large, lovely pond, which attracts great blue herons, egrets, and other wildlife. There are two trails—a 0.25-mile asphalt-paved route and a slightly longer wood-chip version—that take you much closer to the pond. Both pass beautiful wildflower expanses and oak trees. On a recent spring afternoon, I spotted a mated pair of mallard ducks, as well as two Canada geese and their four fluffy goslings. If you don't have time even for a stroll, I recommend seeking out the bench behind the nature center, where you can spend a few minutes soaking in the sights and sounds of the pond. (You can hear, but mercifully not see, nearby street traffic.) Note that no picnicking, bicycles, or pets are allowed, and that the gates close at sunset.

↙ essentials

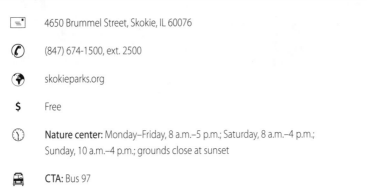

⌸   4650 Brummel Street, Skokie, IL 60076

✆   (847) 674-1500, ext. 2500

🌐   skokieparks.org

$ Free

🕐   **Nature center:** Monday–Friday, 8 a.m.–5 p.m.; Saturday, 8 a.m.–4 p.m.; Sunday, 10 a.m.–4 p.m.; grounds close at sunset

🚌   CTA: Bus 97

peaceful place 31

EVANSTON ART CENTER

Evanston, Northern Suburbs (MAP FIVE)

category ↙ scenic vistas ✪ ✪

*H*oused in a Tudor mansion, the Evanston Art Center sits on a bluff overlooking small Lighthouse Beach on the shore of Lake Michigan. There's plenty to see inside and on the front lawn, including exhibitions of student art and commissioned site-specific sculptures. But the real serenity lies just behind the art center.

There you'll find three wooden benches scattered among a grove of trees. Choose one to perch on, and you'll be treated to the sights and sounds of the lake—splashing waves,

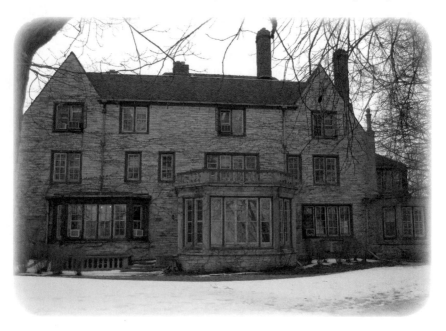

The Evanston Art Center after snowfall

crying gulls, and sighing winds—as well as the nearby historic Grosse Point Lighthouse. Bonus: On the other side of the art center's parking lot sits a playground, while the beach is just a quick walk away. That means that you can park your family (making sure any kids are supervised, of course) in one of those spots while you escape to the benches for a bit. The beach does get noisy on warm afternoons, so time your visit accordingly. One of the most pleasant times to stop by is just before sunset on a summer evening, when your only companions are likely to be a few beachgoers dipping their toes into the waves.

⌣ essentials

✉	2603 Sheridan Road, Evanston, IL 60201
☎	(847) 475-5300
🌐	evanstonartcenter.org
$	Free (gallery suggested donation, $3)
⏱	**Galleries:** Monday–Thursday, 10 a.m.–9 p.m.; Friday–Saturday, 10 a.m.–4 p.m.; Sunday, 1–4 p.m. **Grounds:** Daily, sunrise–sunset.
🚌	**CTA:** Purple Line, Central stop; Bus 201

peaceful place 32

EVANSTON FRIENDS MEETING HOUSE

Evanston, Northern Suburbs (MAP FIVE)

category ↶ spiritual enclaves ✪ ✪ ✪

*W*hether or not you are familiar with the spiritual practices of Friends—more commonly known as Quakers—a visit to a Sunday morning service here will seem extraordinarily peaceful indeed. Rather than a service with hymns, readings, a sermon, and so forth, Quakers simply sit in silence until one of them feels moved to stand up and speak about some spiritual matter. Like other Friends, the Evanston Quakers are very welcoming of visitors and don't press their beliefs on others. However, you don't have to attend a service to benefit from the peacefulness on offer here, thanks to the meetinghouse's large park-like lawn. Especially on weekdays during the school year, when students at the nearby middle school are in class, the lawn offers a place to rest for a spell in a natural setting. Picnic tables invite passersby to bring their lunches, while shady trees and colorful wildflowers provide respite for the eyes. The meetinghouse itself is a pleasant sight too: a redbrick edifice with an arched doorway, it reminds me of a one-room schoolhouse.

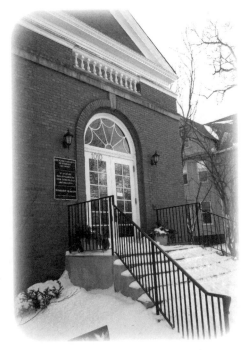

Snowy steps lead to the Evanston Friends Meeting House.

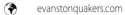 essentials

⊡   1010 Greenleaf Street, Evanston, IL 60202

℃   (847) 864-8511

🌐   evanstonquakers.com

$ Free

🕐   Sunday services: 10 a.m.

🚌   **CTA:** Purple Line, Dempster stop; Bus 201 or 205

peaceful place 33

FERN ROOM, GARFIELD PARK CONSERVATORY

East Garfield Park, West Side (MAP THREE)

category ⌇ parks & gardens ⭐ ⭐

*I*magine a lagoon from a Disney film, complete with trickling waterfalls, lush greenery, cartoon mermaids, and turtles placidly sunning themselves on rocks. Minus the mermaids, that's what the Garfield Park Conservatory's Fern Room resembles. At the same time, this beautiful landscape looks so natural that you'll understand why early visitors to this century-old conservatory suspected that its creators had simply glassed over an existing ecosystem. On the contrary, it was all created by noted

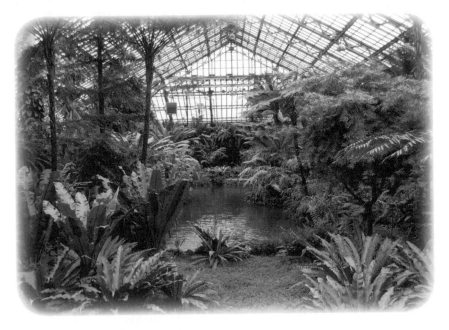

The Garfield Park Conservatory's lush lagoon

landscape architect Jens Jensen in the early 20th century. Jensen's goal was to evoke a prehistoric landscape, and he succeeded; you half expect a brontosaurus to sleepily lift its head above the towering ferns.

I like to meander around the lagoon, pausing near the waterfalls that feed it to spy on the goldfish hovering in the shallows below. The conservatory has a wealth of other offerings, too, such as a children's garden, a horticulture hall with rotating flower shows, and a re-creation of painter Claude Monet's garden at Giverny. But if it's a quiet tropical getaway you're after, the Fern Room is where you'll find it. Note that while it is safe to park at the conservatory or take public transportation there, the surrounding neighborhood is sketchy, so exercise caution.

Sadly, in June 2011, an unusually strong hailstorm shattered more than half of the Fern Room's glass roof, rendering the room unsafe for visitors. At press time, it was closed until further notice. However, portions of the rest of the conservatory remain open. Call or see the conservatory's website for details.

↩ essentials

▤   300 North Central Park Avenue, Chicago, IL 60624

✆   (312) 746-5100

⊕   garfieldconservatory.org

$ Free

🕐   Thursday–Tuesday, 9 a.m.–5 p.m.; Wednesday, 9 a.m.–8 p.m.

🚌   **CTA:** Green Line, Conservatory stop; Bus 20

peaceful place 34

57TH STREET BOOKS

Hyde Park, South Side (MAP FOUR)

category ⌣ reading rooms ✪ ✪

*W*alk down two steps, give the heavy front door a good shove, and you're here—in what is, as I discovered during my days as a student at the nearby University of Chicago, the best of the Hyde Park neighborhood's many bookshops. A spacious front room gives way to a series of smaller enclaves, all packed with well-organized bookshelves and the serious readers they attract. Between the new-paperbacks table, the lavish cookbook selection, the wealth of sci-fi and mystery novels, and the sheaves of indie magazines, it's easy to find something to pore over at the round reading table in the back room.

This is a particularly good place to spend an hour off your feet after a trip to the nearby Museum of Science and Industry, especially if you have children in tow; the children's section here is terrifically well stocked, and if you time things carefully, you can even hit the 10:30 a.m. storybook hour on Wednesday mornings. (You can consider perusing a bit while your tots become enthralled with that entertainment.) That said, the atmosphere here is virtually always conducive to a relaxing browse. Don't be surprised if you find yourself deep in quiet conversation with one of the knowledgeable staff members, or if you discover that he or she is also a graduate student in, say, Russian philosophy or nuclear physics.

⌣ essentials

⌐ 1301 East 57th Street, Chicago, IL 60637

☎ (773) 684-1300   ⦿ semcoop.com

$ Free except for purchases   ◷ Daily, 10 a.m.–8 p.m.

🚌 **Metra Electric District:** 55th-56th-57th Street Station; **CTA:** Bus 55

peaceful place 35

FOURTH PRESBYTERIAN CHURCH

Magnificent Mile, Downtown (MAP ONE)

category ↙ spiritual enclaves ✪ ✪

*R*esting serenely amid the posh shops of the Magnificent Mile, elegant, enormous Fourth Presbyterian makes for a refreshing sight. Its Gothic complex centers on a green courtyard that—though open to Michigan Avenue and its traffic—still manages to emanate a sense of peaceful order. If you just need a quick breather from the hordes on the sidewalk, step into the courtyard for a few moments and admire the stone fountain there. Or, to really saturate yourself in silence, head to the sanctuary entrance at the southwest corner of Michigan Avenue and Delaware Place, and sit down inside.

A cozy experience this is not: enormous stained glass windows flank what seem like acres of numbered wooden pews (enough to seat 1,300 during Sunday services). But if you're looking to swaddle yourself in quiet grandeur, you're in the right place. For those in search of inspirational material, you will find devotional pamphlets and copies of recent sermons in the entryway. Free concerts of classical and religious music take place at noontime on Fridays year-round, or you may stumble upon musicians rehearsing for a service. (I was recently treated to an impromptu clarinet and organ performance.)

↙ essentials

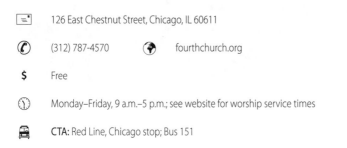

▤	126 East Chestnut Street, Chicago, IL 60611
☎	(312) 787-4570 ⊕ fourthchurch.org
$	Free
⦾	Monday–Friday, 9 a.m.–5 p.m.; see website for worship service times
🚌	**CTA:** Red Line, Chicago stop; Bus 151

peaceful place 36

GOLDEN BEAN, HOTEL INDIGO
Gold Coast, North Side (MAP TWO)
category ⌣ quiet tables ❂ ❂

*T*o find this jauntily decorated coffee-shop-cum-café, just enter the Hotel Indigo and keep walking straight back. At first glance, it might not seem particularly peaceful, what with all the sherbet-colored hues. True, Zen chic this ain't, with zippy green and peach pillows adorning bright-white deck chairs, light fixtures shaped like seashells, and an enormous painting of palm leaves. But the ambience here is as chill as the decor is loud.

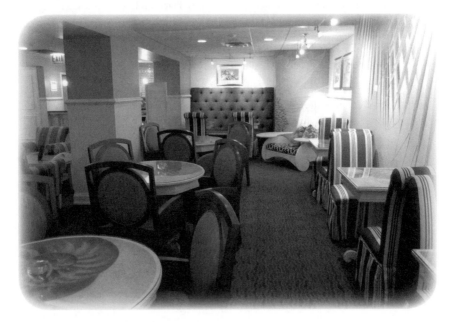

The Golden Bean's lounge makes a quiet reading room.

Especially on weekday mornings and afternoons, when foot traffic in the adjacent lobby slows to a trickle, you're all but guaranteed to have the place to yourself. It helps, too, that the Hotel Indigo sits on the refined Gold Coast, rather than the noisier Magnificent Mile—and that the café is located well away from the hotel's main entrance. Curl up in one of those (very comfortable) deck chairs with a book. Or plop down on a sofa with your smartphone (on the vibrate setting, please). Or sit at one of the tables with a laptop. Regardless, your only disturbance is likely to be the occasional person stopping in for a cup of coffee to go.

⌁ essentials

📧 1244 North Dearborn Parkway, Chicago, IL 60610

📞 (312) 787-4980

🌐 goldcoastchicagohotel.com

$ **Entrées:** $12–$19

🕐 Monday–Friday, 6 a.m.–10 p.m.; Saturday–Sunday, 7 a.m.–10 p.m.

🚌 **CTA:** Red Line, Clark/Division stop; Bus 22

peaceful place 37

GRACELAND CEMETERY

Uptown, North Side (MAP TWO)

category ༄ enchanting walks ✪ ✪ ✪

*G*raceland is less a cemetery than a vast, 150-year-old city of the dead—a place to stroll down leaf-strewn paths among stately tombs, where some of Chicago's most famous historic figures have found their eternal rest. Among the graves here are those of George Pullman (inventor of the railroad car that bears his name), Marshall Field (the department store magnate), and mapmaker Andrew McNally.

But some of the most intriguing tombs belong to lesser-known figures. Consider early settler Dexter Graves, whose resting place is marked with a hooded, menacing, Darth Vader–like statue. To find it, enter at the main gate at the juncture of Clark Street and Irving Park Road. Then follow the main path to the right, and look for the green, life-size figure in the distance. A high wall surrounds the cemetery, blocking the outside world and making it easy to feel as if you've traveled back to Victorian times—except for the occasional rumble of the El and the distant lights of

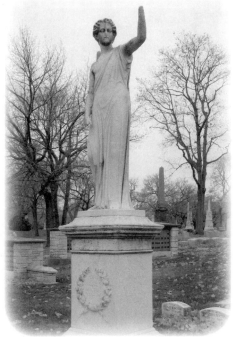

Eerie stone figures dot the landscape of Graceland Cemetery.

Wrigley Field. Tip: Graceland is quite large, and it's easy to find yourself outside eyesight or earshot of other people. Definitely stop at the cemetery office for a map, bring a friend along, and be back at the gate well before closing time. Or make it easy by taking a tour led by the Chicago Architecture Foundation ([312] 922-8687; **caf.architecture.org**).

essentials

4001 North Clark Street, Chicago, IL 60613

(773) 525-1105

gracelandcemetery.org

$ Free

Grounds: Daily, 8 a.m.–4:30 p.m.
Office hours: Monday–Friday, 9 a.m.–4 p.m.; Saturday, 10 a.m.–3 p.m.

CTA: Red Line, Sheridan stop; Bus 22

peaceful place 38

THE GREAT HALL, UNION STATION

West Loop, Downtown (MAP ONE)

category ↙ reading rooms ⊗ ⊗

W hat's the opposite of a peaceful place? With more than 50,000 people treading its corridors and platforms daily, Union Station would seem to be it. Unless, that is, you forgo the station proper for its Great Hall—a massive waiting room with a soaring, five-story skylight.

To find it, enter the building on the west side of Canal Street, directly across from the station's main entrance. You'll find yourself in what feels like a set from a 1920s movie,

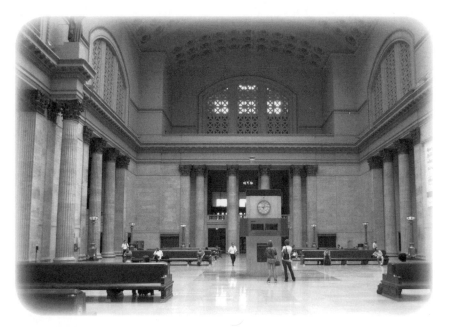

Massive marble pillars hold up Union Station's Great Hall.

and no wonder: some scenes from the Prohibition mobster flick *The Untouchables* were filmed here. The Beaux Arts room features sweeping staircases, Corinthian columns, a marble floor, and banks of curved wooden seats where you can sit and read or write as long as you like. But what you might notice first is the surprising level of quietness. Somehow, cell phone conversations disappear into the space instead of reverberating in it. And, as of 2011, the Great Hall has air-conditioning for the first time, meaning that the AC's gentle whoosh helps muffle ambient noise as well.

⌣ essentials

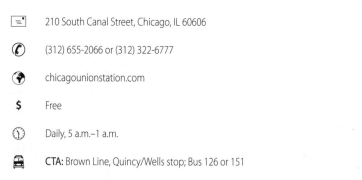

210 South Canal Street, Chicago, IL 60606

(312) 655-2066 or (312) 322-6777

chicagounionstation.com

$ Free

Daily, 5 a.m.–1 a.m.

CTA: Brown Line, Quincy/Wells stop; Bus 126 or 151

peaceful place 39

THE GRIND CAFE

Ravenswood, North Side (MAP TWO)

category ↵ urban surprises ⊗ ⊗

I knew about this tiny, independently owned coffeehouse for years but tended to avoid it—despite its free Wi-Fi and great food—because it can be both noisy and jam-packed. Then a friend clued me in to its secret, near-silent back garden. Not only is it not visible from inside, but no sign alerts customers to its presence. To get to it,

take a deep breath, suppress the feeling that you're going to get in trouble for this, and walk behind the counter and directly through the kitchen to the orange door. Open it, turn right, open a second door, and you're there—in a walled-off sliver of green space with a few small tables, some sun umbrellas, a scattering of wild-flowers, and almost no street noise. Nor can you hear the hubbub in the café. On cloudy or cool days in particular, you're even likely to have the garden all to yourself. There's no table service, so get your coffee and goodies first (I highly recommend the vanilla cupcakes); then settle in for some quiet time.

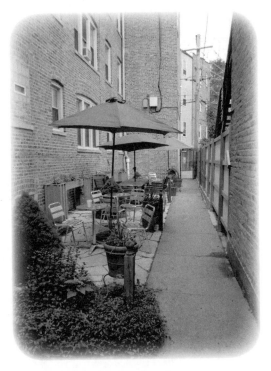

The hidden back patio at the Grind Cafe

⌐ essentials

▭ 4613 North Lincoln Avenue, Chicago, IL 60625

Ⓒ (773) 271-4482

⊕ grindchicago.com

$ **Beverages:** $1.55–$4.50; **salads and sandwiches:** $2.75–$7.25

☾ Monday–Friday, 7 a.m.–8 p.m.; Saturday, 8 a.m.–8 p.m.; Sunday, 8 a.m.–7 p.m.

🚋 **CTA:** Brown Line, Western stop; Bus 11

peaceful place 40

HARPER AVENUE

Hyde Park, South Side (MAP FOUR)

category ↵ enchanting walks ✪ ✪

*O*n this short but calming walk along Harper Avenue, between two of the neighborhood's main drags—57th and 59th streets—you'll pass one interesting home after another. Unlike other residential blocks of Hyde Park, many of which feature little brick apartment buildings, this stretch of the avenue is lined with single-family homes of seemingly every style and color palette.

Look for the purple house with darker purple trim, the yellow house with red trim, and the house that looks as if its painter took inspiration from a Crayola box. The street is particularly pleasant in fall, when the many deciduous trees along the route begin changing color and shedding their leaves—gaily adding to the neighborhood hues. This walk makes for an excellent segue between the Midway Plaisance Readers' Garden (see page 102) or Rockefeller Chapel (see page 153) and 57th Street Books (see page 56), even if it does require a slight detour. Simply walk east along 59th Street until you reach Harper Avenue; then turn left to begin the walk. Upon reaching 57th Street, turn left again and walk four blocks to find the bookstore.

↵ essentials

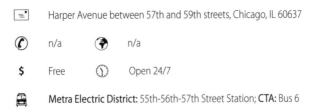

| ▤ | Harper Avenue between 57th and 59th streets, Chicago, IL 60637 |

| ☏ | n/a | ☷ | n/a |

| $ | Free | ☽ | Open 24/7 |

| ⛁ | **Metra Electric District:** 55th-56th-57th Street Station; **CTA:** Bus 6 |

peaceful place 41

HISTORIC PULLMAN LANDMARK DISTRICT
Pullman, South Side (MAP FOUR)
category ↙ historic sites ❂ ❂

For fewer than 20 years, what was touted as "the world's most perfect town," Pullman, Illinois, sat just south of Chicago. Built in the early 1880s by George Pullman, inventor of the railroad sleeping car, this company town boasted beautiful Victorian architecture as well as such modern conveniences as indoor plumbing and garbage pickup. However, after its founder raised rents—but not wages—the town's inhabitants (who were also Pullman's employees) went on strike. In 1907 the town was annexed to the city of Chicago, and its lovely buildings were sold. Happily, many of those buildings have been restored, and tours are available.

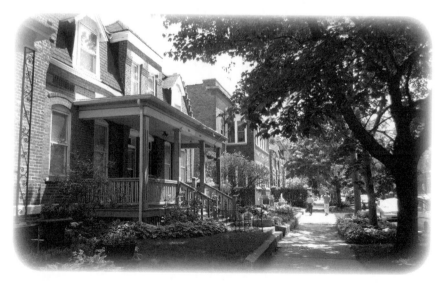

Houses in Historic Pullman are typically red.

The neighborhood's quiet, tree-lined streets and meticulously cared-for homes make a stroll here a calm and pleasant experience. For a self-guided walking tour, pick up a map at the visitor center. (Don't be fooled—the visitor center is not the grand edifice with the clock tower on South Cottage Grove Avenue but rather the nondescript gray building a little farther south on the same street.) If you'd rather learn a little more history, guided walking tours are available on the first Sunday of the month May–October.

⌣ essentials

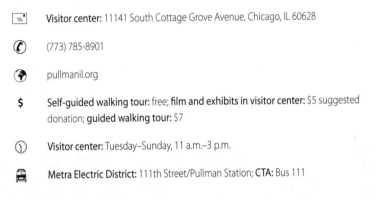

Visitor center: 11141 South Cottage Grove Avenue, Chicago, IL 60628

(773) 785-8901

pullmanil.org

$ Self-guided walking tour: free; film and exhibits in visitor center: $5 suggested donation; guided walking tour: $7

Visitor center: Tuesday–Sunday, 11 a.m.–3 p.m.

Metra Electric District: 111th Street/Pullman Station; CTA: Bus 111

peaceful place 42

HISTORIC WAGNER FARM
Glenview, Northern Suburbs (MAP FIVE)
category ⌣ parks & gardens ✪

*O*nce a real working farm, Wagner Farm is now owned and operated by the Glenview Park District, which treats it mostly as a venue for school-group trips. But who says that adults can't enjoy the sights of cows and chickens too? First thing on weekend mornings, when school groups aren't in attendance and before most families make it there, is the best time to visit for a little bucolic tranquility.

You can stroll the grounds, stopping to see the bustling chicken coop, the little pink pigs in their pen, or the placid black-and-white cows grazing in a green pasture. Afterward, in warm weather, drop into the on-site ice cream shop for a cone; then enjoy it from one of the white rocking chairs out front. If you have kids with you, they can race around the enormous lawn or go inside the visitor center to

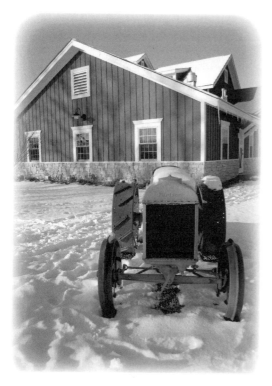

A tractor waiting out the winter at Historic Wagner Farm

do pretend chores such as candling eggs (which entails pressing a button to light up a fake egg to see whether there's a developing chicken inside).

For the cold-tolerant, know that winter here is the quietest time. Even though the animals won't be out and about in inclement weather, you can still walk the grounds and browse around the indoor store, which sells locally made cheese and crafts.

essentials

⌐≡˙⌐   Lake Avenue and Wagner Road, Glenview, IL 60025

📞   (847) 657-1506

🌐   wagnerfarm.org

$ Free

🕐   Monday–Saturday, 9 a.m.–5 p.m.; Sunday, 9 a.m.–3 p.m.

🚌   n/a

peaceful place 43

HOLY WISDOM MONASTERY

Wisconsin, Farther Afield (MAP SEVEN)

category ↙ day trips & overnights ✪ ✪ ✪

*T*he Benedictine Women of Madison may be small in number as, at last count, the community had fewer than five members. But they've created a hugely relaxing retreat center, which lies about a 3-hour drive northwest from Chicago. Open to all, the center sits on 138 acres of restored prairie, through which several walking paths wind (3.8 miles' worth in all). Stroll along one, and you may spot deer grazing or startle a white-tailed rabbit into bounding away through the grass. (Or—as happened to me on one memorable occasion—you may get dive-bombed by a bluebird who thinks you're a little too close to its nest and disturbing its family's peacefulness.)

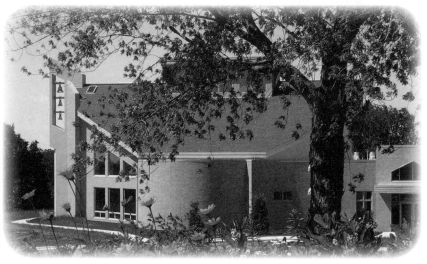

courtesy of Ann Moyer

Holy Wisdom Monastery sits on a restored prairie.

Inside the quiet but welcoming monastery, there's an inviting library, as well as a second-floor sunroom and a small chapel. Visitors can come for the day or stay for a night, a weekend, or longer in plain but comfortable single or double rooms. All are welcome to participate in the community's daily religious services, though no one will be offended if you refrain. I do highly recommend attending the group meals. The food is absolutely delicious and prepared fresh with many local ingredients.

⌣ essentials

✉	4200 County Road M, Middleton, WI 53562
☎	(608) 836-1631
🌐	benedictinewomen.org
$	**Day use:** $36; **room:** $50–$62
🕒	**Day use:** Daily, 8 a.m.–4:30 p.m.
🚍	n/a

peaceful place 44

INDIANA DUNES NATIONAL LAKESHORE

Indiana, Farther Afield (MAP SEVEN)

category ⤴ day trips & overnights ✪ ✪

*W*hen you live in the third most populous city in the United States, it's easy to feel as if the concrete jungle is closing in on you. That's why it's important— no, imperative—to occasionally hop into the car or onto the train and get the heck out. And one of the easiest escapes is the Indiana Dunes, a national lakeshore that lies only about 1 1/2 hours' drive east from Chicago.

The dunes have it all: swimming, hiking, biking, bird-watching, fishing, boating, horseback riding, and picnicking. But your best bet for a peaceful experience is to avoid the summer sunbathing and camping crowds. (For one thing, as attractive as the

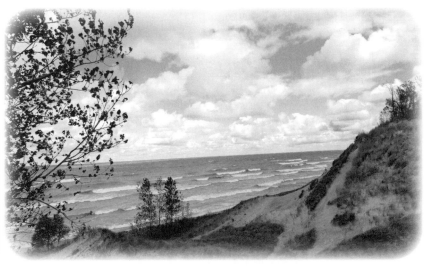

The dunes provide a perfect outlook on the sights of Lake Michigan.

beach is, swimming can be treacherous here, thanks to a plethora of rip currents and a paucity of lifeguards.)

Instead, choose a more offbeat activity such as hiking the moderately difficult 3-mile Inland Marsh Trail or, weather permitting, snowshoeing the 6.4-mile Ly-co-ki-we Trail. If you visit between March and May, be sure to seek out the Heron Rookery on the River Trail to see great blue herons returning to their nests for the season.

↙ essentials

🖃	Visitor center: 1215 North State Road 49, Porter, IN 46304
🕻	(219) 926-7561
🌐	nps.gov/indu
$	**West Beach area:** $6 per car per day; **campsites:** $15 per night; otherwise, free
🕐	**Visitor center:** Summer hours, daily, 8 a.m.–6 p.m. Winter hours, daily, 8:30 a.m.–4:30 p.m. **Trails:** Daily, 7 a.m.–sunset
🚍	**Chicago South Shore and South Bend Railroad:** Miller, Portage/Ogden Dunes, Dune Park, or Beverly Shores stations

peaceful place 45

INTERNATIONAL MUSEUM OF SURGICAL SCIENCE

Gold Coast, North Side (MAP TWO)

category ⌇ museums & galleries ✪ ✪

*O*ne of Chicago's lower-profile museums, the International Museum of Surgical Science is also one of its quietest. While the exhibits may not be considered classically peaceful and are not an experience for the queasy, they are engaging enough to transport you from modern-day concerns.

Housed in a historical mansion overlooking Lake Shore Drive are four floors of fascinating medical artifacts. Some are tied to a specific scientific innovation, such as the very lancet used by Edward Jenner to administer the first smallpox vaccine. Others simply

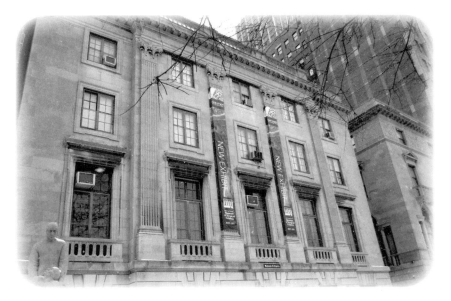

The great stone face of the International Museum of Surgical Science

evoke the medical realities of a particular era, such as the amputation saw from 16th-century Austria and the trepanning instruments from the Incan empire.

The museum also hosts rotating special exhibits, such as "Our Body: The Universe Within," which showcases the human body via actual, meticulously preserved corpses. If you're intent on soaking up all the medical knowledge you can and have time to spare, purchase the audio tour. Otherwise, I enjoy simply strolling along the museum's Italian marble floors and through its high-ceilinged rooms, pausing periodically to examine whatever artifact catches my eye. Either way, I've never encountered more than a few other visitors, and I know that I can count on this destination for some quiet time.

↙ essentials

📧   1524 North Lake Shore Drive, Chicago, IL 60610

📞   (312) 642-6502

🌐   imss.org

$ Adults: $10–$22; students and military members with ID and seniors age 65 and older: $6–$16; children ages 4–13: $6–$12; children age 3 and younger and museum members: free; Tuesdays: free

🕐   Tuesday–Friday, 10 a.m.–5 p.m.; Friday–Saturday, 10 a.m.–9 p.m.; Sunday, noon–5 p.m. (last admission 1 hour before closing)

🚌   **CTA:** Red Line, Clark/Division stop; Bus 22

peaceful place 46

INTUIT: THE CENTER FOR INTUITIVE AND OUTSIDER ART

River West, West Side (MAP THREE)

category ↙ museums & galleries ✪ ✪

*A*s its name suggests, this small but intriguing gallery in the West Town neighborhood is devoted to intuitive and outsider art—works produced by people who are not part of the mainstream art world. To me, the most charming aspect of a visit here is the opportunity to get to know the artists through the biographical placards that accompany their works.

For example, there's Emery Blagdon, a farmer who lost both parents and three siblings to cancer, and then spent the rest of his life creating wire sculptures he called "healing machines." And then there's the former Folsom Prison inmate–turned-artist who signed his works "Backward Jesus."

All the art here is housed in just two galleries, but I find myself so taken with these curious works that I can easily

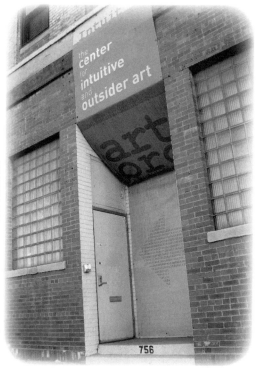

courtesy of Intuit: The Center for Intuitive and Outsider Art

The entrance to Intuit

spend an hour or more just absorbing them. Best of all, I can do so free of the clamor that often accompanies a visit to larger museums. Other visitors to Intuit seem to be after the same quiet, contemplative experience that I seek.

⌣ essentials

| ⊟ | 756 North Milwaukee Avenue, Chicago, IL 60642 |

| 📞 | (312) 243-9088 |

| 🌐 | art.org |

| $ | **Adults and children age 12 and older:** $5; **children age 11 and younger:** free |

| 🕐 | Tuesday–Wednesday and Friday–Saturday, 11 a.m.–5 p.m.; Thursday, 11 a.m.–7:30 p.m. |

| 🚌 | **CTA:** Blue Line, Chicago stop; Bus 66 |

peaceful place 47

ISTRIA CAFÉ

Hyde Park, South Side (MAP FOUR)

category ⌣: quiet tables ❂ ❂

*S*ome people find that a cluttered atmosphere sets their minds free. To me, it's the opposite—how can anyone think with all that mess lying around? Maybe it's for people like me, then, that this café housed in the Hyde Park Arts Center chose its clean, streamlined look. White walls; stainless steel dome lamps; simple armless, cushioned chairs—aah. That sound you hear just may be your visual cortex relaxing. It helps that the clientele here consists largely of one of the quietest segments of the population, namely, graduate students with laptops and deadlines. Then, too, Istria lies a fair distance from the University of Chicago campus, meaning that it's a serious study spot rather than a chatty hangout for students on their way to and from class. If you find yourself restless despite all this serenity (too much espresso?), just ask someone to keep an eye on your computer and go for a wander in the Arts Center galleries for a bit. Or do what I do and settle your soul with one of the excellent gelato flavors.

⌣: essentials

▣   5030 South Cornell Avenue, Chicago, IL 60615

C   (773) 324-9660

⊕   istriacafe.com

$ **Coffee and tea:** $2–$3.50; **gelati:** $3–$5

🕐   Monday–Friday, 6:30 a.m.–7 p.m. (until 9 p.m. in summer); Saturday, 7 a.m.–7 p.m.; Sunday, 7:30 a.m.–7 p.m.

🚌   **Metra Electric District:** 51st-53rd Street Station; **CTA:** Bus 146, 6, and X28

peaceful place 48

JANE ADDAMS HULL-HOUSE MUSEUM
University Village, West Side (MAP THREE)
category ⌁ historic sites ✪ ✪

*M*any small museums, it must be said, fall into the twin traps of overstuffing and under-labeling their exhibits. If you've ever found yourself staring at a heap of ostensibly historic detritus without a clue as to its significance, you know what I mean. Happily, the Jane Addams Hull-House Museum isn't one of these. The curators have done a masterful job of interpreting Addams's legacy of social reform, and they've done so in the very mansion where she lived and worked.

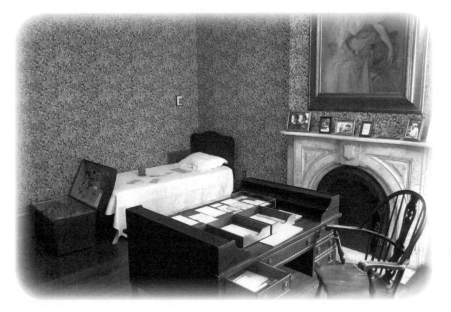

Jane Addams's bedroom

Here you can not only read about Addams's tireless efforts to help the poor but also see historic items that bring them to life—such as the note Addams received from an 11-year-old child pleading for help, or the sewing machine like the kind that impoverished immigrants used during long, exhausting factory days.

Upstairs, you'll see Addams's own bedroom, which includes a display of her Nobel Peace Prize medal (she was the first American woman to win it). It's all available to be enjoyed in relative quiet—and for free. By the way, there's no truth to the bizarre and long-standing rumor that Hull House is haunted by a devil baby, so please make your visit peaceful for everyone by not asking the staff about it.

↙ essentials

▤ 800 South Halsted Street, Chicago, IL 60607

☎ (312) 413-5353

🌐 hullhousemuseum.org

$ Free

🕐 Tuesday–Friday, 10 a.m.–4 p.m.; Sunday, noon–4 p.m.

🚌 **CTA:** Blue Line, UIC-Halsted stop; Bus 8

peaceful place 49

JUDY ISTOCK BUTTERFLY HAVEN, PEGGY NOTEBAERT NATURE MUSEUM

Lincoln Park, North Side (MAP TWO)

category ᨺ urban surprises ✪

*W*ithin the Peggy Notebaert Nature Museum, there's a warm, peaceful getaway beckoning when the Chicago cold reaches oppressive levels. In this tropical atmosphere flit hundreds of butterflies with names as exotic as their appearances— white peacock, painted lady, red cracker, and pink-spotted cattleheart. You will also keep company with the occasional bird, such as the jewellike red-legged honeycreeper or the adorable button quail.

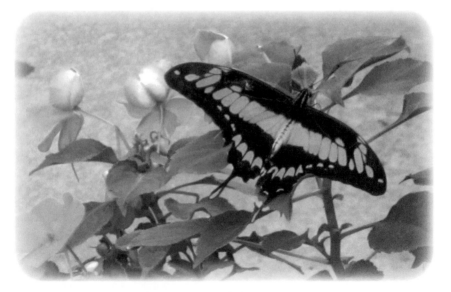

A giant swallowtail taking a breather in the butterfly haven

Greenhouse windows let in sunlight, and hanging vegetation provides a beautiful backdrop for the fluttering creatures. Look for butterflies sitting in sunny spots with their wings open; they're allowing the warmth to raise their body temperature, which is the same as that of the surrounding air. Scattered benches allow you to sit still and enjoy both the sounds of the haven's waterfall and the sights that surround you.

After you exit, be sure to stop for a look at the display of chrysalides. If you're lucky, you'll see a newly created butterfly emerging from one, drops of liquid falling from its wings as it slowly opens and closes them.

The haven is popular with school groups, so to ensure the quietest experience, aim to visit first thing on a Sunday morning.

ᴗ essentials

2430 North Cannon Drive, Chicago, IL 60614

(773) 755-5100

naturemuseum.org

Adults: $9; **students and seniors:** $7; **children ages 3–12:** $6; **children age 2 and younger:** free

Monday–Friday, 9 a.m.–4:30 p.m.; Saturday–Sunday, 10 a.m.–5 p.m.

CTA: Red Line, Fullerton stop; Bus 151

peaceful place 50

JULIUS MEINL

Ravenswood, North Side (MAP TWO)

category ◡: quiet tables ✪

*O*ne of only three U.S. outposts of this Austrian chain (each of them, oddly enough, is in Chicago, and one is a patisserie), Julius Meinl brings an old-world touch to American coffee culture.

In lieu of jumbo muffins and blended iced-coffee drinks, you'll find slices of apple strudel and cups of Vienna Eiskaffee (espresso poured over vanilla ice cream). Even plain old herbal tea gets the full treatment here: instead of a paper cup, you'll receive an individual glass teapot, a china cup and saucer, a small glass of water, and a spice cookie, all served on a silver tray. (I like the orange-ginger tisane, which is an unexpectedly brilliant pink.)

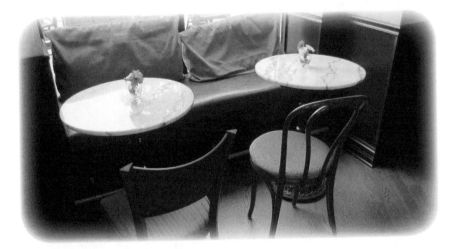

A cozy window seat at Julius Meinl coffeehouse

In other words, this is a place to sit and savor a lovely moment, not to grab a cup of joe and go. Individual blooms in glass vases grace each table, and the padded window seats invite cozying up, especially on a chilly day. This is the quieter of Julius Meinl's two Chicago coffeehouse locations (the other being in the Lake View neighborhood, at 3601 North Southport), but for the most peaceful experience, I still recommend visiting on a weekday midafternoon to avoid the morning and evening rushes.

✍ essentials

4363 North Lincoln Avenue, Chicago, IL 60618

(773) 868-1876

meinl.com

$ Pastries: $2.50–$6.50; **coffee and tea:** $1.70–$4.50

Monday–Thursday, 6 a.m.–10 p.m.; Friday, 6 a.m.–midnight; Saturday, 7 a.m.–midnight; Sunday, 7 a.m.–10 p.m.

CTA: Brown Line, Montrose stop; Bus 11

peaceful place 51

KEMPF PLAZA

Lincoln Square, North Side (MAP TWO)

category ✌ parks & gardens ✪

A few factors combine to make this small brick-paved square (officially named Kempf Plaza but frequently called Giddings Plaza) an appealing place to spend some quiet moments. The stretch of North Lincoln Avenue that forms its western edge is narrow and one-way, making traffic sounds minimal, and splashing water in the square's tiered fountain further masks noise. Metal benches beneath leafy trees make an ideal place to spoon into a cup of something sweet from the adjacent Paciugo gelato shop. And the elaborate metal Lombard Lamp (a gift from the city of Hamburg, Germany), with its garland-toting cherubs, lends a stately, old-fashioned air to the surroundings.

All that said, the local chamber of commerce sponsors outdoor concerts here on some

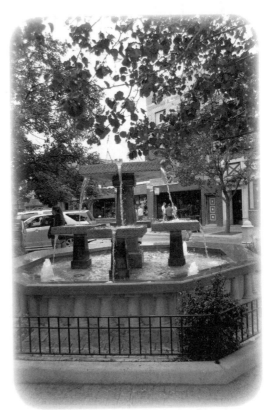

A fountain burbles in Lincoln Square's Kempf Plaza.

summer evenings, and at any time you may encounter a few moms desperate to let their toddlers work off some energy by chasing pigeons around the square. But in general, the weekday atmosphere here is peaceful and pleasant. For added quiet, combine your visit with a trip to The Book Cellar (see page 20) just across the street.

essentials

Giddings Street at Lincoln Avenue, Chicago, IL 60625

Lincoln Square Chamber of Commerce: (773) 728-3890

lincolnsquare.org

$ Free

Open 24/7

CTA: Brown Line, Western stop; Bus 11

peaceful place 52

LADD ARBORETUM

Evanston, Northern Suburbs (MAP FIVE)

category ⤳ outdoor habitats ✪ ✪

*H*ear the word *arboretum,* and you likely picture an isolated, forestlike area with trails and footbridges. The Ladd Arboretum, in contrast, occupies just 17 acres, measures just 0.25 mile wide, and sits between busy McCormick Boulevard and the North Shore Channel canal. Despite its centralized location, the arboretum offers a pocket of peace with its walking paths, flowering trees, and wildflowers.

For the quietest experience, head for the walking path on the canal side, the one that leads behind the on-site Evanston Ecology Center. A bit northeast of the center, you'll

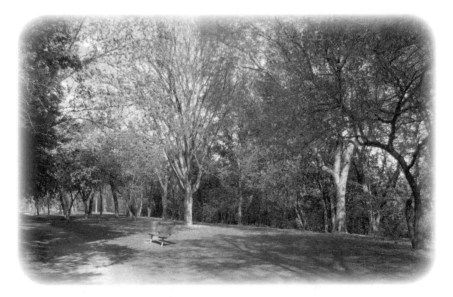

Walking paths thread Evanston's Ladd Arboretum.

find a small waterfall with benches, where you can sit beneath a shady bower and listen to the burble and splash of the water. This is the arboretum's Grady Bird Sanctuary, so keep an eye out for the occasional warbler or waxwing.

As you continue on the path, look for oak, maple, birch, nut, and other trees. For the most dramatic wildflower show, visit in June, when the local blooms reach their peak. If you'd like to learn more about the flora and fauna that make their home here, the Ecology Center offers ongoing nature programs such as one titled Canoe the Canal and another called Backyard Bees.

⌣ essentials

✉ 2024 McCormick Boulevard, Evanston, IL, 60201

☎ (847) 448-8256

🌐 evanstonenvironment.org

$ Free; **nature programs:** $4–$40

🕐 **Arboretum:** Daily, sunrise–sunset.
Evanston Ecology Center: Monday–Friday, 8:30 a.m.–5 p.m.
Also open Labor Day–Memorial Day on Saturdays, 9 a.m.–4:30 p.m.

🚌 **CTA:** Purple Line, Noyes stop;
Metra Union Pacific: North Line, Evanston Central Street Station

peaceful place 53

LAKE FOREST CEMETERY
Lake Forest, Northern Suburbs (MAP FIVE)
category ↲ enchanting walks ✪ ✪ ✪

*T*hough much smaller than Graceland (see page 60) or Rosehill (see page 157) cemeteries, Lake Forest's version is equally beautiful and beguiling in its own way. Fewer historic figures are buried in Lake Forest than at its more famous counterparts in the city, true. But visitors will still enjoy the parklike atmosphere, as well as the numerous unusually designed headstones here. Those include representations of a mother frolicking with her children, a life-size stag, an angel crouching in the grass, and a cleft rock with a dove flying out.

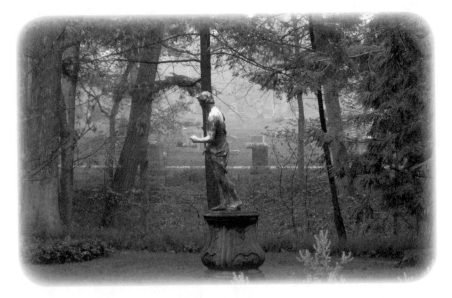

The cemetery's parklike landscape welcomes visitors.

You can drive or walk the paved cemetery paths; either way, you'll pass through the Barrell Memorial Gate—a monument to an only son who drowned nearly 100 years ago—at the cemetery's entrance. One of my favorite things about a walk here is that the cemetery never feels claustrophobic or creepy. Perhaps that is thanks to its location on a bluff overlooking Lake Michigan, or to the banks of daffodils and flowering trees that grace the grounds. Near the entrance, look for the Memorial Gardens, where benches allow you to sit and rest, read, or just think for a spell. Note that the address below will lead you to the cemetery office, which is open by appointment only. To enter the cemetery itself (at 1525 North Lake Road), head to the nearby intersection of Spruce Avenue and Lake Road.

essentials

▤ 520 Spruce Avenue, Lake Forest, IL 60045

✆ (847) 615-4341

🌐 cityoflakeforest.com/cu/bldg/bldg_cem.htm

$ Free

🕐 **May–September:** Daily, 8 a.m.–8 p.m.
October–April: Daily, 8 a.m.–4:30 p.m.

🚆 **Metra Union Pacific:** North Line, Lake Forest Station

peaceful place 54

LINCOLN PARK CONSERVATORY
Lincoln Park, North Side (MAP TWO)
category ↝ parks & gardens ✪ ✪

*O*n a cold day in Chicago—and there's certainly no shortage of them—this small conservatory near the Lincoln Park Zoo promises a brief tropical escape. The glasses-fogging humidity in here is enough to make you entirely forget the blustery outdoors for a bit. The sugarcane, bird-of-paradise, and coffee plants, as well as orange, guava, and banana trees, will only add to your weather amnesia.

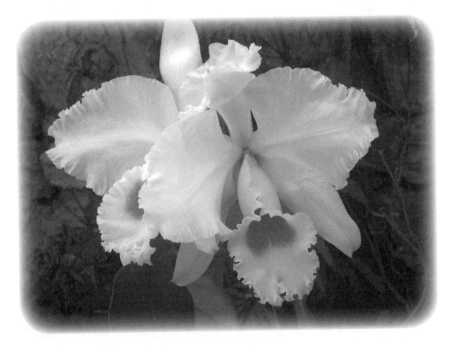

The Lincoln Park Conservatory is abloom year-round.

The first sight upon entering is one of the most stunning: a pond filled with day-blossoming blue water lilies and shining goldfish. Look hard enough and you might find the resident frog. If you become tempted to touch the enormous brown gourdlike objects hanging from a nearby tree, don't. With apologies to Jack Nicholson in *A Few Good Men*, you can't handle the fruit. Those brown things are sausage tree fruit, and they're more fragile than they seem. Skirt them on your way to the quiet Fern Room or the perfumed Orchid House. If you have children in tow, the Orchid House is a must-see, not as much for the flowers as for the koi pond, where the enormous fish swim with their round mouths opening and closing in search of food above the water's surface. The conservatory is open every single day of the year, making it a wonderful place to escape for a few quiet moments on holidays.

essentials

▤	2391 North Stockton Drive, Chicago, IL 60614
✆	(312) 742-7736
⊕	chicagoparkdistrict.com
$	Free
◷	Daily, 9 a.m.–5 p.m.
🚌	**CTA:** Red Line, Fullerton stop; Bus 22

peaceful place 55

LONGWOOD DRIVE DISTRICT

Beverly, South Side (MAP FOUR)

category ↲ enchanting walks ✪ ✪

*W*arning: Walking through this architecturally rich area may make you jealous—not necessarily of the palatial homes, but of the fact that bicyclists and in-line skaters in this neighborhood can actually *coast down a hill.* For the scenic Longwood Drive District, built on a glacial ridge as it is, represents the highest point in famously flat Chicago. (That said, there's no need to pack your hiking boots—this is still an easy stroll.)

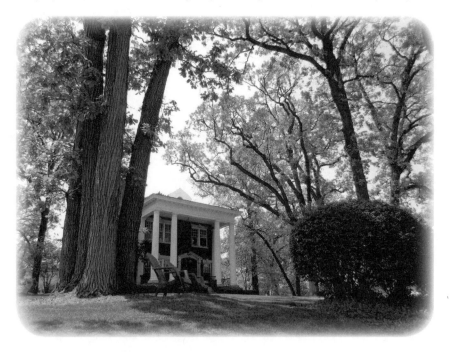

The Longwood Drive District is the home of Chicago's highest point.

Begin in the 9800 block of South Longwood Drive, and proceed south to the 11000 block. You'll pass homes in a bouquet of architectural styles, including examples of Queen Anne, Prairie School, Italianate, and other types. Be sure to keep an eye out for the Givens Castle at 10244 South Longwood Drive. Built as a home in 1886, it's said to be haunted, even now that it's occupied by a Unitarian church. Many of the homes are set back far from the street, and their wide lawns, along with the relatively small amount of traffic on Longwood, lend a pleasantly subdued air to the neighborhood.

essentials

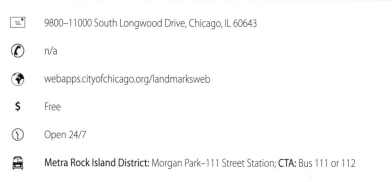

9800–11000 South Longwood Drive, Chicago, IL 60643

n/a

webapps.cityofchicago.org/landmarksweb

Free

Open 24/7

Metra Rock Island District: Morgan Park–111 Street Station; **CTA:** Bus 111 or 112

peaceful place 56

LUTZ CAFÉ

Ravenswood, North Side (MAP TWO)

category ⌣ quiet tables ✪ ✪

A rich pastry, a cup of something hot, and a quiet dining room are often all I need to rejuvenate. But in the age of chatter-filled coffee shops, these magic ingredients can be hard to find. Fortunately, the Lutz Café has been offering all three since 1948, when a husband and wife who emigrated from Europe set up shop here to peddle cakes, strudels, and other confections. The café also sells actual meals, but it's hard to keep your mind on savories once you spot the case of sweets standing right by the front door.

Choose one of the several small vase-topped tables, and ask for the Vienna coffee service. Here is what will come to you on a silver tray: a cup of coffee served with whipped cream, plus the pastry of your choice—perhaps a slice of Black Forest cake or strawberry whipped-cream torte. Particularly on weekdays, when the café is least busy, you'll likely be able to savor this combination in peace, with only the occasional talkative group of grandmas to interrupt the quiet. In summer, a back garden allows diners to eat al fresco.

⌣ essentials

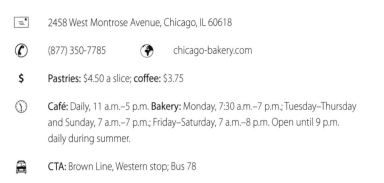

🖃	2458 West Montrose Avenue, Chicago, IL 60618
☎	(877) 350-7785 🌐 chicago-bakery.com
$	**Pastries:** $4.50 a slice; **coffee:** $3.75
🕓	**Café:** Daily, 11 a.m.–5 p.m. **Bakery:** Monday, 7:30 a.m.–7 p.m.; Tuesday–Thursday and Sunday, 7 a.m.–7 p.m.; Friday–Saturday, 7 a.m.–8 p.m. Open until 9 p.m. daily during summer.
🚌	**CTA:** Brown Line, Western stop; Bus 78

peaceful place 57

MADONNA DELLA STRADA CHAPEL

Rogers Park, North Side (MAP TWO)

category ⌁ spiritual enclaves ✪ ✪ ✪

*J*ust adjacent to Lake Michigan on the campus of Loyola University sits an Art Deco jewel: the Madonna della Strada, or "Our Lady of the Way," Chapel. Serving as the main university chapel, the 70-plus-year-old Madonna della Strada underwent an interior renovation in 2006–2007. Its many treasures include a new pipe organ, a fountainlike baptismal font, richly colored stained glass windows of the saints, and painted icons galore. The golden color used in many of the icons lends a warm, appropriately heavenly air to the chapel's interior. The chapel is open daily 7 a.m.– 7 p.m., and as long as you are respectful of your surroundings, no one minds if you wander around to examine the paintings and statuary.

I must recommend that you visit the Madonna shrine at the front of the church, to the right as you face the altar. I literally gasped the first time I saw it. Thousands of

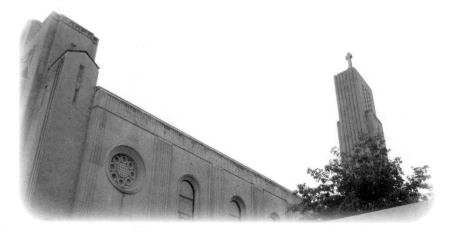

The chapel of Our Lady of the Way anchors Loyola University's Rogers Park campus.

tiny blue and gold mosaic tiles, banks of white orchids and blue candles, a portrait of a serene, crowned Virgin Mary with the Christ Child—it inspires awe even among the not remotely devout. Unless you happen upon a worship service (see below for days and times), your only company will be the occasional additional visitor or two.

⌣ essentials

✉ 1032 West Sheridan Road, Chicago, IL 60660   ☎ (773) 508-8045

🌐 luc.edu/sacramental_life/Madonna_Della_Strada_Chapel.shtml

$ Free

🕐 Daily, 7 a.m.–7 p.m. **Masses:** Sunday, 10:30 a.m., 5 p.m., and 9 p.m.; Monday–Thursday, noon and 5:15 p.m.; Friday, noon. **Masses in summer:** Sunday, 10:30 a.m.; Monday–Friday, noon. See website for additional worship service times.

🚌 **CTA:** Red Line, Granville stop; Bus 151

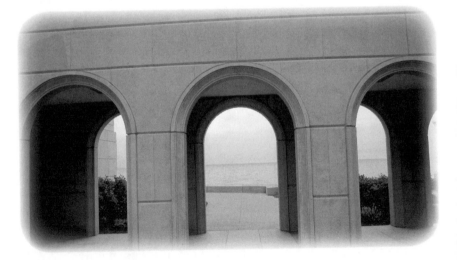

The chapel of Madonna della Strada overlooks Lake Michigan.

peaceful place 58

MARY BARTELME PARK

West Loop, West Side (MAP THREE)
category ✨ parks & gardens ✪ ✪

*T*his is one of the newest city parks in Chicago—and it shows. Bartelme Park (also known as Adams & Sangamon Park, after its nearest intersection) opened in 2010 to rave reviews, including one from *Chicago Tribune* architecture critic Blair Kamin.

If you suspect by now that Mary Bartelme Park consists of much more than the usual square of grass and tiny playground, you're right. Visitors enjoy not only a large, sophisticated play area for children but also a sunken, fenced-off dog exercise space. But peacefulness seekers, not to worry: what I like best about this artfully created park are the grassy mounds that provide a sense of separation between the noisier areas and the quieter ones.

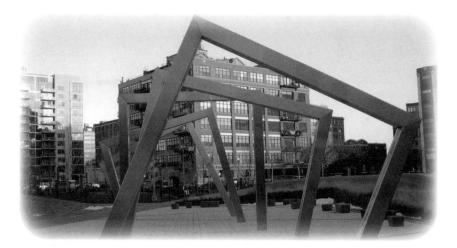

The entrance gates at the park double as misting fountains on hot days.

There's much here for someone in search of beauty and quiet: the dramatically curving landscape features native plant life, and a series of intentionally askew stainless steel arches emits refreshing clouds of mist during the summer months. And if you climb the tallest mound, you'll take in a sensational view of the downtown skyline, including the Willis Tower.

⌣ essentials

☑	115 South Sangamon Street, Chicago, IL 60607
☎	(312) 746-5962
🌎	chicagoparkdistrict.com (in the list of parks, search for "Bartelme, Mary")
$	Free
🕐	Daily, sunrise–sunset
🚍	**CTA:** Blue Line, UIC-Halsted stop; Bus 8

peaceful place 59

MAY T. WATTS READING GARDEN, MORTON ARBORETUM

Lisle, Western Suburbs (MAP SIX)

category ↵ outdoor habitats ✪ ✪ ✪

etting to the Morton Arboretum from the city requires a bit of effort, true. In traffic, it can take a full hour to drive here from downtown. But your diligence will be more than rewarded. Founded by Joy Morton of the famous Morton Salt Company, the 1,700-acre arboretum harbors a breathtaking array of trees (fitting, since Morton's father founded Arbor Day). Also on-site are 16 miles of trails, 11 gardens (including a 1-acre hedge maze), two ponds, five lakes, and lots of opportunities to hike, bike, ski, or even snowshoe.

All that said, if you find yourself needing an escape within an escape, visit the less commonly frequented May T. Watts Reading Garden. A small walled garden, it sits immediately adjacent to the arboretum's Sterling Morton Library, not far from the main visitor center. There you can enjoy the sounds of a trickling fountain while you park yourself on a bench under a leafy pergola with the book of your choice. In spring, look for snowdrops among the garden's foliage; in warmer weather, you might see hostas or orange coneflowers. The walls that surround the garden mean that you'll be pleasantly secluded from other arboretum visitors.

↵ essentials

⌨ 4100 Illinois Route 53, Lisle, IL 60532

☏ (630) 968-0074   ✪ mortonarb.org

$ **Adults:** $11 ($7 on Wednesdays); **seniors age 65 and older:** $10 ($6 on Wednesdays); **children ages 2–17:** $8–$11 ($5 on Wednesdays)

☼ Daily, 7 a.m.–sunset   🚗 n/a

peaceful place 60

MIDWAY PLAISANCE READERS' GARDEN

Hyde Park, South Side (MAP FOUR)

category ↵ outdoor habitats ✪

*L*ocated on the Midway Plaisance, a narrow, mile-long park that connects Washington Park and Jackson Park between 59th and 60th streets, the Readers'

Garden takes its name from the pastime generally enjoyed on the many benches that dot the site. In pleasant weather, they're the perfect spot to relax with a book. Look for the garden on the northern side of the Midway between Ellis and Woodlawn avenues. You will see that the space centers on a massive statue of Carl von Linné (also known as Linnaeus), the Swedish botanist who created the scientific classification of plant and animal species. That is something to think about as you watch one of the garden's resident *Sylvilagus floridanus* (cottontail rabbits) bounce by.

Unfortunately, depending on the time of day, the many

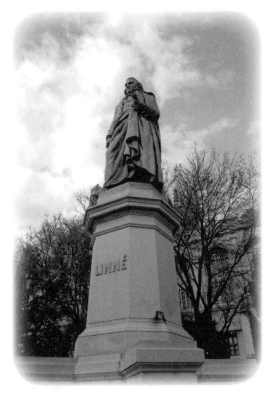

A statue of Swedish botanist Carl Linnaeus looms over the garden.

University of Chicago undergraduates who use the garden as a shortcut between the main campus and 60th Street can make the setting a little less serene. In that case, I suggest abandoning your bench for an eastbound walk along the handy paved path, which is bordered by trees, shrubbery, and bushes.

essentials

⌨ 59th Street between Ellis and Woodlawn avenues, Chicago, IL 60637

📞 (312) 745-2470

🌐 chicagoparkdistrict.com

$ Free

🕐 Open 24/7

🚍 **Metra Electric District:** 59th Street–University of Chicago Station; **CTA:** Bus 59

peaceful place 61

MONTROSE HARBOR

Uptown, North Side (MAP TWO)

category ↲ scenic vistas ✪ ✪

*F*irst, the good news: Montrose Beach has a reputation as one of the quietest and least-crowded stretches of sand in Chicago. Now the better news: The lakefront along Montrose Harbor, on the opposite side of the peninsula where the beach lies, is even quieter and even less crowded. True, you'll have to swap lying on the sand for stretching out on the grass or walking along a concrete path. But the solitude factor makes that an easy trade.

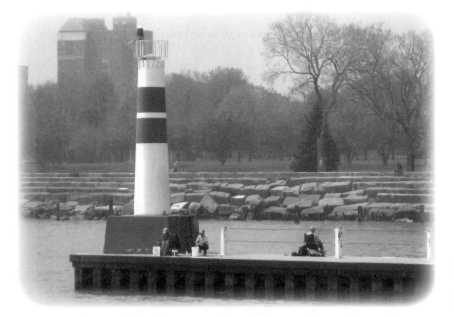

Waiting for a nibble at Montrose Harbor

Close to the west end of the harbor, you'll find a number of shaded benches. If you, like me, consider it strangely relaxing to just sit and watch docked boats bobbing in the water, this is the spot for you. Otherwise, follow Montrose Harbor Drive to the lakefront side of the harbor. From here you can see not only the Chicago skyline but also seagulls perpetually wheeling overhead, sailboats catching the wind, and a few people placidly fishing. Swimming isn't allowed, but nothing is stopping you from sitting barefoot on the edge of the pier to catch lake breezes wafting up from below—or from spreading a towel out on the nearby grass to catch a few rays.

⌣ essentials

▣   601 West Montrose Drive, Chicago, IL 60613

✆   (312) 742-7527

🌐   chicagoharbors.info/harbors/montrose.php

$ Free

🕑   Daily, 6 a.m.–11 p.m.

🚌   **CTA:** Red Line, Wilson stop; Bus 78 or 81

peaceful place 62

MUSEUM OF CONTEMPORARY ART CHICAGO
Streeterville, Downtown (MAP ONE)
category ⌁ museums & galleries ✪ ✪

*C*hicago's Museum of Contemporary Art stands on the former site of a National Guard armory. But there's nothing bellicose about this beautiful streamlined temple of art, devoted to works created since 1945. After ascending the enormous staircase at its main entrance, you'll find a constantly rotating collection of sculptures, paintings, photographs, and film installations. Especially on weekdays, the atmosphere is serene, so no one is likely to derail your train of thought as you contemplate works such as Jeff Koons's *Rabbit* (a metallic form of a faceless bunny) or Claes Oldenburg's *Sculpture in the Form of a Fried Egg* (what it sounds like).

When you're done perusing, treat yourself to lunch at the museum's restaurant, Puck's at the MCA, which offers sweeping views of Lake Michigan. Or just go for a stroll in the outdoor terraced sculpture garden. It's worth, too, stopping in the gift shop, where you can choose

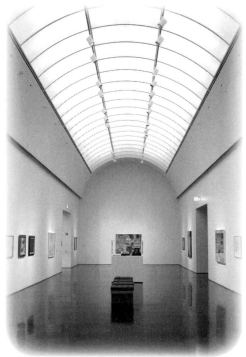

MCA gallery installation © 2011 Museum of Contemporary Art, Chicago

A quiet gallery at the Museum of Contemporary Art Chicago

among such wonderfully weird items as a birdhouse shaped like a geodesic dome, the world's smallest solar-powered car, and a coatrack made of coat hangers.

⌣ essentials

⊟   220 East Chicago Avenue, Chicago, IL 60611

ⓒ   (312) 280-2660

🌐   mcachicago.org

$ **Adults:** $12; **students with ID and seniors:** $7;
    **museum members, military, and children age 12 and younger
    (accompanied by adult):** free;
    Illinois residents: free on Tuesdays

🕐   Tuesday, 10 a.m.–8 p.m.; Wednesday–Sunday, 10 a.m.–5 p.m.

🚌   **CTA:** Red Line, Chicago stop; Bus 147 or 151

peaceful place 63

MUSEUM OF CONTEMPORARY PHOTOGRAPHY

The Loop, Downtown (MAP ONE)
category ↙ museums & galleries ✪ ✪

This tiny museum on the Columbia College campus provides a sense of calm far out of proportion to its size. With an emphasis on photographs taken since 1936, the works that hang in the museum's rooms are mostly landscapes, both rural and urban. Some of them are by well-known names such as Alfred Eisenstadt and Ansel Adams, others by talented up-and-comers. Two of my favorites are Dorothea Lange's *Toward Los Angeles, California* and Jay Wolke's images of Chicago's Dan Ryan Expressway. A subset of the overall collection is devoted to contemporary works by photographers from the Midwest.

The compact first floor is quiet enough, but climb the stairs to the even smaller second and third floors to encounter a near-silent atmosphere in which to soak in the works. The third floor also offers tables and chairs for reading and studying, as well as a computer station where you can browse the museum's entire collection. Not only is the museum peaceful, but it's also free. Note that because the museum closes whenever Columbia College closes, and also when new exhibits are being installed, it's wise to check the museum's website before your visit.

↙ essentials

✉ 600 South Michigan Avenue, Chicago, IL 60605

☎ (312) 663-5554   🌐 mocp.org $ Free

🕐 Monday–Wednesday and Friday–Saturday, 10 a.m.–5 p.m.; Thursday, 10 a.m.–8 p.m.;
    Sunday, noon–5 p.m.

🚌 CTA: Red Line, Harrison stop; Bus 3 or 147

peaceful place 64

MUSIC BOX THEATRE

Lake View, North Side (MAP TWO)

category ⌣ historic sites ⭐

$\mathcal{N}$ ot everyone thinks of going to the movies as a peaceful activity, particularly if your local cinema features sticky floors and shrieking children along with its coming attractions. But in this 1920s-era theater, moviegoing becomes an almost serene experience if you time your visit carefully.

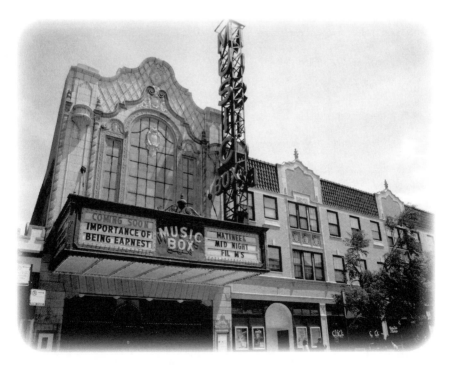

The historic Music Box shows both classic and modern movies.

I recommend weekend mornings, when classic films along the lines of *Vertigo* and *Chinatown* are shown; that's when the audience consists of true movie buffs, and the atmosphere is most amenable to the serious cinematic experience. Aside from the films themselves, the main auditorium is the draw here. Twinkling lights, which suggest stars, sparkle in the arched, dark-blue ceiling, and old-fashioned red-velvet curtains part dramatically to expose the movie screen. Live organ music accompanies silent movies, and— perhaps most thrilling of all—the snack bar puts real butter on the popcorn. If you're willing to sacrifice your quiet for the sake of some fun, visit around the winter holidays, when the theater traditionally shows a double feature of *It's a Wonderful Life* and *White Christmas*, interspersed with group carol-singing.

◡ essentials

▣   3733 North Southport Avenue, Chicago, IL 60613

☏   (773) 871-6604

🌐   musicboxtheatre.com

$ $9.25 (with daily matinee and all-day Monday discounts)

🕐   See website for showtimes.

🚌   **CTA:** Brown Line, Southport stop; Bus 9

peaceful place 65

NAPERVILLE RIVERWALK

Naperville, Western Suburbs (MAP SIX)

category ↜ enchanting walks ❂ ❂

*A*ttention, Chicagoans who think that there's nothing more to the suburbs than strip malls and chain restaurants: think again. Since its creation in 1981, Naperville's beautiful, serene riverwalk has epitomized the best of the 'burbs—quiet, lush, and low-key. Stretching nearly 2 miles alongside the west branch of the DuPage River, it winds through well-tended parks, over green hills, and near splashing fountains. Three covered bridges, a carillon (also known as a bell tower), multiple plazas, and an

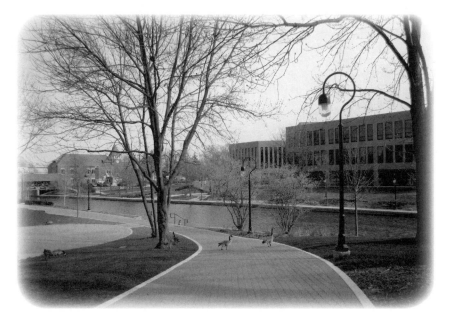

A brick-lined path leads along the Naperville Riverwalk.

outdoor amphitheater add to the scenery. In warm weather, you can rent a four-passenger paddleboat or go in-line skating here too. Naperville's nearby downtown makes it easy to buy an ice cream cone or soda to take along on your stroll. Have kids in tow? Take them to the playground that sits along the riverwalk just west of Centennial Beach. Or just let them (futilely) chase the many mallard ducks and Canada geese that frequent the area. A free parking lot located near the corner of Washington Street and Jackson Avenue makes it easy to leave your car without fuss.

⌣ essentials

▧   320 West Jackson Avenue, Naperville, IL 60540   📞   (630) 305-5984

🌐   napervilleriverwalk.com $ Free   🕙   Daily, 6 a.m.–midnight

🚌   **Metra Burlington Northern Santa Fe (BNSF) Railway:** Naperville Station

A charming covered bridge along the Naperville Riverwalk

peaceful place 66

NATURE BOARDWALK, LINCOLN PARK ZOO
Lincoln Park, North Side (MAP TWO)
category ↜ enchanting walks ✪ ✪

$\mathcal{A}$s one of the very few remaining free zoos in the country, Lincoln Park Zoo is frequently jam-packed with families, particularly when the weather is nice. That means that, as intriguing and educational as the animal exhibits are, visiting here isn't always a tranquil encounter. Happily, as of 2010, the zoo offers a quieter experience: strolling the new Nature Boardwalk around South Pond.

The 0.5-mile walk offers chances to see turtles, toads, wood ducks, and other water-friendly creatures in their natural habitat. Because they're not the charismatic mega-fauna

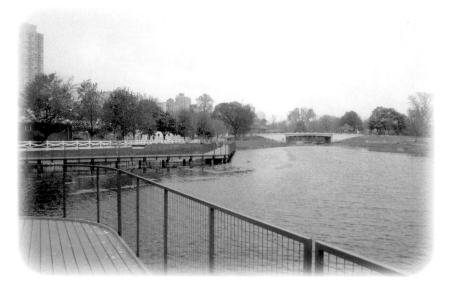

The Nature Boardwalk winds for 0.5 mile around South Pond.

that draw big crowds elsewhere in the zoo, you're guaranteed a more serene, yet fascinating, viewing experience. As you pass under the bridge that spans the boardwalk, look up and you might spy swallows building their nests in the slats. Look, too, for endangered black-crowned night herons, which stop on an island within the pond during their seasonal migrations. When you're done with your stroll, you can reward yourself with an ice cream cone at the Patio at Café Brauer, which sits adjacent to the boardwalk.

essentials

⌨   2001 North Clark Street, Chicago, IL 60614

☎   (312) 742-2000

🌐   lpzoo.org

$ Free

🕐   Daily, 6 a.m.–11 p.m.

🚌   **CTA:** Red Line, Fullerton stop; Bus 22

peaceful place 67

NOBLE TREE COFFEE & TEA
Lincoln Park, North Side (MAP TWO)
category ⌣ quiet tables ❂ ❂

REE WIFI. GREAT COFFEE. SERIOUS PIE. That is what the sign proclaims outside this Lincoln Park house-turned-coffee-shop. For my money, the owners should think about adding "serious silence" to that tagline, for, despite the playful ambience (think orange fireplace and trompe l'oeil sky on the ceiling), Noble Tree's patrons seem more interested in quietly reading or working than in chattering or kibitzing. And the three floors of seating allow you to easily get away from the espresso-machine noise behind the counter.

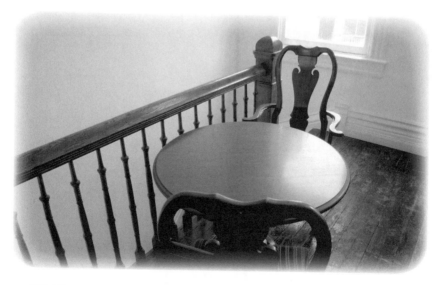

Third-floor getaway at Noble Tree Coffee & Tea

On the second and third floors, you'll find comfortable leather club chairs and large windows, with background music that's audible but laid-back. In the summer, an outdoor patio provides additional seating (albeit in a less quiet atmosphere, as the coffee shop sits on busy Clark Street near several other businesses). A tasty bonus: Noble Tree's menu includes items from Chicago's own Metropolis Coffee and Hoosier Mama Pie Co. *Note:* To access the free Wi-Fi, you'll need to ask for a code when you make a purchase, and the code is good for a 2-hour stretch.

↶ essentials

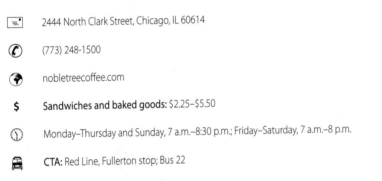

2444 North Clark Street, Chicago, IL 60614

(773) 248-1500

nobletreecoffee.com

$ Sandwiches and baked goods: $2.25–$5.50

Monday–Thursday and Sunday, 7 a.m.–8:30 p.m.; Friday–Saturday, 7 a.m.–8 p.m.

CTA: Red Line, Fullerton stop; Bus 22

peaceful place 68

NOMI KITCHEN

Magnificent Mile, Downtown (MAP ONE)

category ⌒ quiet tables ✪ ✪

or the most peaceful breakfast just off the Magnificent Mile, head to NoMI Kitchen, the recently remodeled seventh-floor restaurant of the Park Hyatt Hotel. And for the most magnificent views of downtown, arrive as early as possible and ask to be seated at one of the coveted window-side tables. At this hour, the prices are cheaper, the dress code is looser (nice jeans are fine), the dining room is at its quietest, and the service is just as impeccable as at dinner.

The menu offers well-executed classics with a twist, such as buttermilk pancakes topped with strawberry-rhubarb compote and ricotta cheese; buckwheat crêpes with smoked salmon, lemon crème fraîche, dill, and capers; and Maine lobster Benedict with citrus hollandaise. Or keep things light and healthy with one of the seasonal smoothies, made with the usual juices and soy milk as well as the much-less-usual spinach leaves, cocoa powder, and aloe vera. One tip: When you enter the hotel lobby, look for the elevator discreetly labeled NOMI across from the concierge desk; it goes directly to the seventh floor.

⌒ essentials

▤	Park Hyatt Hotel, 800 North Michigan Avenue, Chicago, IL 60611
☏	(312) 239-4030
⊕	nomirestaurant.com
$	**Breakfast entrées:** $9–$22
⊙	**Breakfast:** Monday–Friday, 6:30–10:30 a.m.; Saturday, 7–11 a.m.; Sunday, 7–10:30 a.m.
⛟	**CTA:** Red Line, Chicago stop; Bus 147

peaceful place 69

NORTH PARK VILLAGE NATURE CENTER

North Park, North Side (MAP TWO)

category ↙ enchanting walks ✪

*D*eer, in the middle of the city? Yes. Just off one of the city's busiest byways, Pulaski Road, more than 40 deer roam about 155 acres of unspoiled forest, prairie, and wetland. It's far from unusual to come across these gentle creatures, alone or in groups, while you're strolling along one of the several walking trails here. You may also spot foxes, rabbits, and—if you perfect your sighting skills by attending one of the special evening programs led by naturalists—owls. Check out a pair of binoculars and a field guide from the nature center staff to up your chances of identifying any wildlife you encounter.

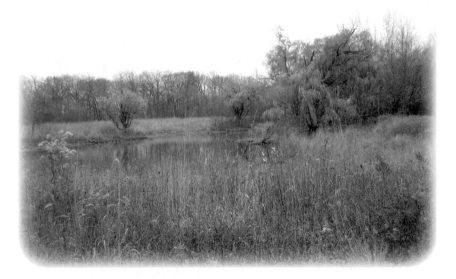

Prairie grasses border a pond at the nature center.

To fully escape from the city, avoid the north end of the nature preserve, where views of nearby traffic may interfere with your reverie. Elsewhere, the setting is almost completely blocked by tall maple, oak, and other trees, and the sound of the wind sighing through tall grasses acts as Mother Nature's form of white noise. After a bracing walk outdoors, it's fun to browse the nature center's educational displays, and I particularly recommend the live honeybee exhibit.

essentials

📧 5801 North Pulaski Road, Chicago, IL 60646

📞 (312) 744-5472

🌐 chicagoparkdistrict.com

$ Free

🕐 Daily, 10 a.m.–4 p.m.

🚌 **CTA:** Bus 53 or 84

peaceful place 70

NORTH POND

Lincoln Park, North Side (MAP TWO)

category ⌣ quiet tables ✪ ✪

*F*or super-stressed couples, simply going out to dinner can feel like a secret getaway. North Pond's hidden location—a renovated ice skaters' warming shelter within Lincoln Park—takes that sense of escape to the next level. To find the restaurant, go to the corner of Lakeview and Deming streets (where, by the way, the restaurant's valet service is located); then take the walking path east into the park. A few minutes' walk

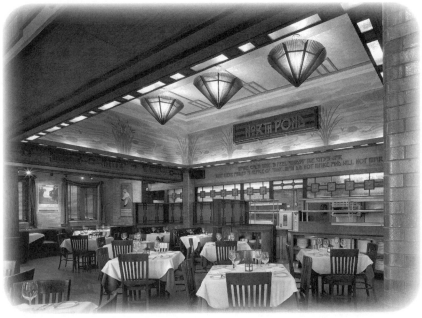

courtesy of Garrick Peterson

North Pond's interior features an Arts and Crafts theme.

brings you to the restaurant, which sits poised on the shore of the pond from which it takes its name. You'll feel as if you've come across a private oasis, particularly when you taste the seasonal, as-local-as-possible ingredients on which the chef relies. One recent favorite comes to mind: half-moons of pasta filled with roasted squash and cheese and served with grilled leeks, bourbon cranberries, and candied pecans.

Dine during the day for spectacular views of the pond, or in the evening for a heightened sense of snugness and escape. In colder months, maximize the cozy factor by asking to be seated near the front room's fireplace.

✍ essentials

⊟ 2610 North Cannon Drive, Chicago, IL 60614

ⓒ (773) 477-5845

🌏 northpondrestaurant.com

$ **Entrées:** $32–$38; **seasonal tasting menu:** $85 per person

🕐 Tuesday–Thursday and Sunday, reservations accepted from 5:30 p.m. (last reservation at 8:30 p.m.); Friday–Saturday, reservations accepted from 5:30 p.m. (last reservation at 9:15 p.m.); **Sunday brunch:** 10:30 a.m.–1:30 p.m. Note that North Pond is closed on Tuesdays January–April.

🚌 **CTA:** Red Line, Fullerton stop; Bus 22 or 151

peaceful place 71

OAK PARK PUBLIC LIBRARY (MAIN LIBRARY)
Oak Park, Western Suburbs (MAP SIX)
category ⌇ reading rooms ✪ ✪ ✪

etween the ubiquitous banks of public-use computers and the frequent hordes of schoolkids, it can be surprisingly difficult to find a little peace and quiet in many urban libraries. One delightful exception is Oak Park's main library, which feels almost like an unusually hushed upscale café. (As of June 2011, in fact, eating is permitted in many areas of the library. Ask a staff member for details.)

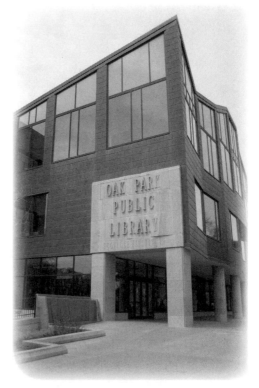

Look for the posted map that demarcates the library by green, yellow, and red spaces. Green means that talking and cell phone conversations are acceptable in that area, yellow indicates that only whispering and texting are OK, and red means that no talking or cell phone use is permitted. In search of absolute quiet? Head to the silent reading room on the third floor.

But no matter what space you choose, you'll find truly comfortable chairs for lounging, cheerful

The exterior of Oak Park's main library

mobiles of blue and green glass, and large windows overlooking adjacent Scoville Park. For that matter, the park itself makes for a pleasant bout of solitude, with tidy beds of tulips and walking paths that twist over and around a central hill.

☿ essentials

✉	834 Lake Street, Oak Park, IL 60301
☎	(708) 383-8200
🌐	oppl.org
$	Free
🕐	Monday–Thursday, 9 a.m.–9 p.m.; Friday, 9 a.m.–6 p.m.; Saturday, 9 a.m.–5 p.m.; Sunday, 1–6 p.m.
🚌	**CTA:** Green Line, Oak Park stop

peaceful place 72

OLD EDGEBROOK HISTORIC DISTRICT

Edgebrook, West Side (MAP THREE)

category ↙ enchanting walks ✪ ✪ ✪

*I*n 1894 Edgebrook was created as a railroad suburb, a peaceful neighborhood removed from the city proper but connected to it via a nearby train station. In the century following, it became even more peaceful once the Cook County Forest Preserve acquired much of the land surrounding it. This neighborhood is now tucked so far into the trees that only two small streets connect it to the rest of the city.

Oddly for a Chicago neighborhood, its streets have no curbs, lending it a small-town ambience. Adding to the neighborhood's character, the houses here are of myriad designs, including bungalow, Colonial Revival, and Queen Anne. There are no businesses in Edgebrook (unless you count the adjacent golf course), so a stroll around the neighborhood feels purely rural and residential. Do take heed of the many deer-crossing signs! On a recent visit, I spotted no fewer than five deer sauntering across the streets. Particularly around twilight, keep a sharp eye out as you drive, and remember that if one bounds across your car's path, at least one more is likely to follow in a moment.

↙ essentials

✉	West Devon and North Caldwell avenues, Chicago, IL 60646
☎	(773) 631-2854
🌐	webapps.cityofchicago.org/landmarksweb
$	Free
🕐	Open 24/7
🚌	**Metra Milwaukee District:** North Line, Edgebrook Station; **CTA:** Bus 84

peaceful place 73

THE ORIENTAL INSTITUTE MUSEUM
Hyde Park, South Side (MAP FOUR)
category ⌣ museums & galleries ✪ ✪ ✪

he only noise in this museum is the soft whoosh of the climate-control system, making for an atmosphere so quiet that you'll see the occasional visitor just sitting and reading a book on a bench. Thousands of artifacts from the world's oldest civilizations are on display in this museum on the campus of the University of Chicago. Jewelry,

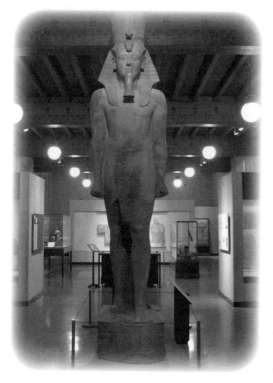

letters, toys, pottery, and other items from everyday life blend with more spectacular objects, such as Egyptian mummies and a 14-foot, human-headed winged bull statue from Iraq.

The most dramatic moment in any visit here comes when you turn the corner out of the Megiddo Gallery, at which point you'll be suddenly confronted with a 17-foot statue of King Tutankhamen (otherwise known as King Tut). You'll likely spend some time entranced by the fact that he looks powerful and graceful at the same time. I also love the delicate, vibrant pendants of

An ancient statue seems to stride through the Oriental Institute.

lapis lazuli, silver, and carnelian from 2900–2350 BC in the Mesopotamian section. By offering self-guided audio tours and signage that's both engaging and explanatory, the curators have done a wonderful job interpreting the displays for the public. Afterward, if you have any gifts to buy, the gift shop overflows with jewelry inspired by pieces from ancient times.

↙ essentials

✉ 1155 East 58th Street, Chicago, IL 60637

☎ (773) 702-9514

🌐 oi.uchicago.edu/museum

$ **Adults and children age 12 and older:** $7 suggested donation; **children age 11 and younger:** $4 suggested donation; cash only

🕐 Tuesday and Thursday–Saturday, 10 a.m.–6 p.m.; Wednesday, 10 a.m.–8:30 p.m.; Sunday, noon–6 p.m.

🚌 **Metra Electric District:** 59th Street–University of Chicago Station; **CTA:** Bus 6 or 55

peaceful place 74

OSAKA JAPANESE GARDEN, JACKSON PARK

Hyde Park, South Side (MAP FOUR)

category ↙ parks & gardens ✪ ✪ ✪

*L*ike many of Chicago's most beautiful attractions, the Osaka Japanese Garden has its roots in the 1893 World's Columbian Exposition, the Chicago fair that commemorated the 400th anniversary of Christopher Columbus's voyage to the New World. During the exposition, a Japanese temple and garden were created in this area. Unfortunately, they fell into disrepair over the centuries, and the temple was destroyed by arson shortly after World War II. Happily, the garden has since been restored, and a beautiful teahouse has been added.

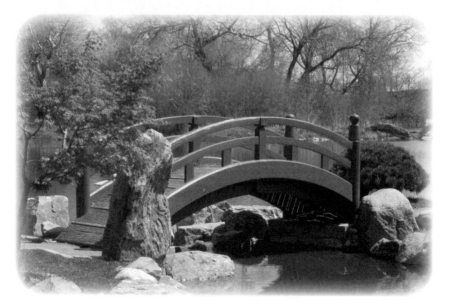

A traditional curved bridge graces the Osaka Japanese Garden.

The easiest way to find it is to drive to the Museum of Science and Industry (see page 42), go to the farthest parking lot behind the museum, and look for the small orange signs reading JAPANESE GARDEN. Follow them, and park your car. A 10-minute walk will take you to the garden, with its winding paths, waterfall, bonsailike trees, pond, covered wooden bridge, and stone lanterns. The garden is part of the Paul Douglas Nature Sanctuary, meaning that you are likely to see a wealth of birdlife (in addition to a wealth of visitors wearing binoculars around their necks). Still, as birders want peace and quiet as much as you do, this is a situation not likely to challenge the reason you came here.

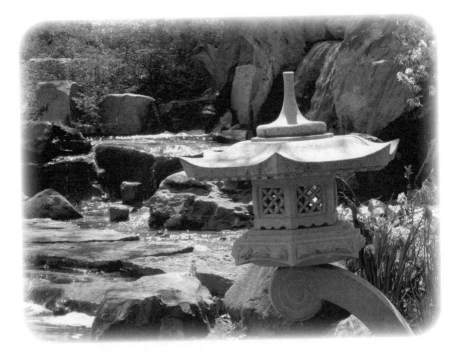

A stone lantern rests beside the garden's trickling waters.

⌣ essentials

⌨ Behind Museum of Science and Industry in Jackson Park
(6401 South Stony Island Avenue, Chicago, IL 60637)

✆ (773) 256-0903

🌐 hydepark.org/parks/osaka2.htm

$ Free

🕐 Daily, 6 a.m.–11 p.m.

🚌 **Metra Electric District:** 55th-56th-57th-Street Station;
CTA: Bus 2, 6, 10, or 55

peaceful place 75

OUR LADY OF SORROWS BASILICA

East Garfield Park, West Side (MAP THREE)

category ⌣ spiritual enclaves ✪ ✪ ✪

*Y*ou might be tempted, as you approach this Italian Renaissance–style church, to linger just outside it, in the manicured prayer garden—the one with the benches and angel sculptures. But traffic noise from the nearby busy intersection, along with the slightly run-down character of the surrounding neighborhood, will urge you inside, where the real contemplative experience awaits.

If the doors are locked, ring the bell at the adjacent monastery, and someone will show you into the sanctuary. Prepare to gasp: the basilica's domed ceiling, adorned with hundreds of carved roses, seems to enfold you like the cloak of a saint. I love to slowly stroll the sanctuary's perimeter (when Mass isn't being held, of course) to peer into the

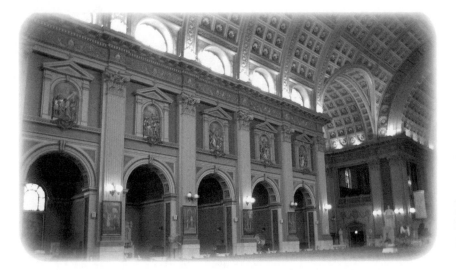

The basilica's lavish interior

ten side chapels. The most beautiful to my eyes is that of Our Lady of Fatima, where a white-robed Virgin Mary stands on a sky-blue cloud, worshipped by children and lambs. To the left of the high altar, look for a sign pointing you to the dimly lit Pieta Chapel, where you can sit and contemplate a replica of Michelangelo's famous sculpture. The basilica lies only about a 5-minutes' drive from the Garfield Park Conservatory (see page 54), so why not combine your visits for a really peace-infused day?

⌇ essentials

✉️   3121 West Jackson Boulevard, Chicago, IL 60612

📞   (773) 638-0159   🌐   ols-chicago.org $ Free

🕐   Monday–Friday, 9 a.m.–4:30 p.m.; Saturday, 9 a.m.–noon; Sunday, 7:30 a.m.–noon. Check website for Mass times.

🚌   **CTA:** Blue Line, Kedzie-Homan stop; Bus 52 or 126

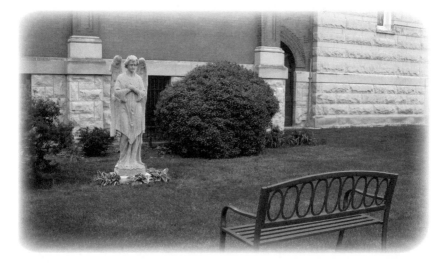

Prayer garden outside the basilica

peaceful place 76

THE PALM COURT, DRAKE HOTEL

Streeterville, Downtown (MAP ONE)

category ⌣ quiet tables ✪ ✪

*W*henever I walk into the venerable Drake Hotel, I automatically think of words ending in "sh," such as *posh, lush, shush,* and *hush.* Blame it on the so-deep-it-muffles-sound carpet, maybe. Or perhaps just on the reputation of its afternoon tea, which is served in the Palm Court lounge, as a serenely elegant, supremely filling experience.

Teatime here meets that description, for sure, but don't be intimidated. You can enjoy a quiet moment at the Drake Hotel even if you're not: a) wearing a large, beflowered hat, or b) prepared to put away an entire plate's worth of pastries. I visited recently in search of nothing more than a lemonade and was politely greeted and seated despite my blue jeans.

Much of the ambience here comes from the splashing of the restaurant's fountain and from the live harp music. Together, they manage to keep the lounge feeling mellow even when every table is filled. Reservations are recommended, especially in chillier weather, when a cup of hot Lapsang souchong tea or Earl Grey tea sounds most appealing.

⌣ **essentials**

✉	140 East Walton Place, Chicago, IL 60611		
☏	(312) 787-2200	✈	thedrakehotel.com
$	**Afternoon tea:** $35 per person	☼	Daily, 1–5 p.m.
🚌	**CTA:** Red Line, Chicago stop; Bus 3, 145, or 147		

peaceful place 77

PALMISANO (STEARNS QUARRY) PARK
Bridgeport, South Side (MAP FOUR)
category ↵ parks & gardens ✪ ✪

*I*mmediately upon entering Palmisano Park—one of the city's newest—you have a decision to make: up or down? Follow the paved slope up the hill to your left, and you'll be rewarded with a fantastic view of the Chicago skyline on one side, the houses of the Bridgeport neighborhood on the other. Follow the flat walking path to your right, descend the stairs to the fishing pond, and you'll find a bank of ancient dolomite limestone, formed so long ago that dinosaurs weren't even walking the earth yet. Or, if you insist, just stay on terra firma and enjoy the sight of the metal fountain near the entrance;

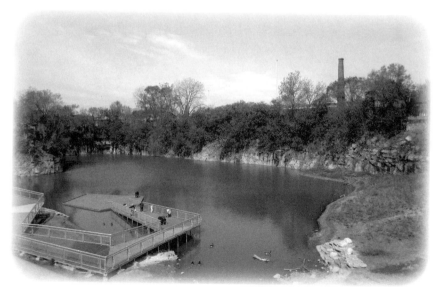

A quarry turned fishing pond at Palmisano Park

it was designed to mimic the shape of the cranes that worked this site when it was still a quarry. Some noise from nearby traffic can be heard, but at least it's forced to compete with the songs of the many birds in the park, which include downy woodpeckers, blue jays, sapsuckers, and more. Wherever you roam here, keep your eyes open for the tiny fossils that you may spot in the park's limestone boulders.

essentials

✉	2700 South Halsted Street, Chicago, IL 60608
☎	(312) 742-7529
🌐	chicagoparkdistrict.com
$	Free
🕐	Daily, 8 a.m.–7 p.m.
🚌	**CTA:** Orange Line, Halsted stop; Bus 8

peaceful place 78

THE PARK AT LAKESHORE EAST

The Loop, Downtown (MAP ONE)

category ↶ parks & gardens ✪ ✪

*E*ven on a balmy day, I've encountered only a few other park-goers here. That is a mystery, as this is one of the most beautiful and relaxing green spaces to be found in all of downtown Chicago. I especially recommend it as a getaway from noisy, chaotic Michigan Avenue.

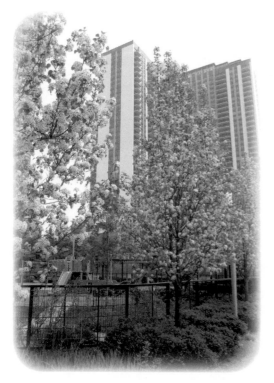

A gated playground is among the draws at the Park at Lakeshore East.

To locate it, simply head east on Randolph Street from Michigan, turn left on North Field Boulevard, and walk a block. When you come to the descending staircase, you're there. Walk down the steps, and you'll find a grassy 6-acre expanse threaded by walking paths, edged by fountains, and dotted by flowering trees. Look for crabapple, redbud, and pear trees, among others. An enclosed dog park and separate children's play area make it easy to amuse any small companions you've brought along. Traffic sounds are minimal, thanks to the luxury high-rises that loom on each side of the park, and any noise that does arise is muted by the splashing of the fountains. After sundown, the fountains are lit to provide a pleasing twilight display. When you're ready to head back to the hustle and bustle and want a lift, there are usually cabs aplenty waiting nearby (thanks to those high-rises I mentioned).

◡ essentials

⊡ Bounded by East South Water Street, North Westshore Drive, East Benton Place, and North Park Drive, Chicago, IL 60601

☏ n/a   ⊕ magellandevelopment.com/lakeshore-east/park

$ Free   ⏰ Daily, 6 a.m.–11 p.m.

🚌 **CTA:** Brown Line, Randolph/Wabash stop; Red Line, Lake stop; Bus 147

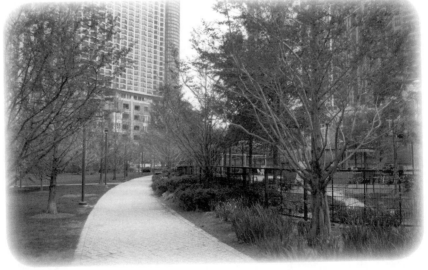

Paved walking paths thread the park.

peaceful place 79

LA PETITE FOLIE
Hyde Park, South Side (MAP FOUR)
category ⌣ quiet tables ❁ ❁

rench food in a strip mall may seem like a *petite folie* (little madness) in itself. But this restaurant's Cordon Bleu–trained chef, delicious dishes, affordable prices, and whisper-quiet dining room add up to very sane reasons to come here, indeed.

For the most serene experience, visit at lunchtime on a weekday, when only a few other diners will be in evidence and when the waitstaff can devote their full attention to you. The restaurant's heavy carpet muffles noise beautifully, making a meal here an entirely shout-free experience even when the dining room is full. As for the menu, I favor the creamy, warming chicken-and-mushroom crêpes or one of the simple luncheon omelets. Word has it that the Alsatian onion tart is exquisite, but I have not yet sampled it. For dessert, the amply portioned crème brûlée arrives flecked with vanilla bean and finished with a caramel crust.

Peaceful parking happens to be one of the easiest aspects of this delightfully easy experience: it's free, it's nearby, and it's ample in the Hyde Park Shopping Center's on-site lot. You'll have no meter to feed, no valet to tip, and no parallel parking to accomplish.

⌣ essentials

🖃 1504 East 55th Street, Chicago, IL 60615

☏ (773) 493-1394   🌐 lapetitefolie.com $ Entrées: $15–$25

🕓 Tuesday–Friday, 11:30 a.m.–2 p.m. and 5 p.m.–closing;
    Saturday–Sunday, 5 p.m.–closing

🚊 **Metra Electric District:** 55th-56th-57th Street Station; **CTA:** Bus 55

peaceful place 80

PING TOM MEMORIAL PARK

Chinatown, South Side (MAP FOUR)

category ↙ parks & gardens ✪ ✪

I made regular noshing and shopping pilgrimages to Chinatown for years before I discovered this beautiful, off-the-beaten-track park. You'll find its entrance at the corner of 19th and Wells streets. (Or, for much of the year, you can get there by taking a boat ride on the river, thanks to the delightful Chicago Water Taxi service; see **chicago watertaxi.com** for fares and schedule.) Situated in a former railroad yard along the Chicago River, the park features not only a charming riverwalk lined with weeping willows but also well-tended banks of daffodils and azaleas, as well as scenic views of downtown. You'll have a particularly good vantage point for taking in the Willis Tower. Surprisingly little traffic noise floats down from the nearby 18th Street Bridge,

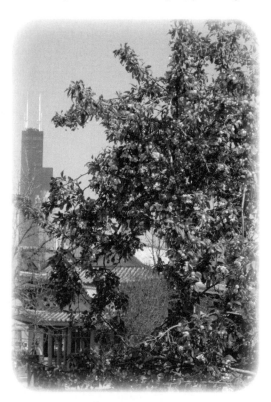

A view of Willis Tower from Ping Tom Memorial Park

but you will hear the occasional rumble of the El as it cranks by. A fenced-off playground at one end of the park attracts plenty of small fry, but if you want to escape their cheerful noise, it's easy enough to head to the area far opposite. At lunchtime, I highly recommend bringing a picnic of takeout dim sum from the nearby Phoenix Restaurant (2131 South Archer Avenue; [312] 328-0848; **chinatownphoenix.com**).

↵ essentials

⊟ 300 West 19th Street, Chicago, IL 60616

© (312) 746-5962

🌐 chicagoparkdistrict.com

$ Free

🕓 Daily, 7 a.m.–10:30 p.m.

🚌 **CTA:** Red Line, Chinatown stop; Bus 62

peaceful place 81

P.O.S.H.

River North, Downtown (MAP ONE)

category ↝ shops & services ✪

*I*f you're shopping for a one-of-a-kind gift, dislike the noisy chain stores of nearby North Michigan Avenue, or both, you can't do better than to step into this small boutique. Whatever the season in Chicago, here you'll encounter "April in Paris" or one of the other equally charming vintage tunes that always seem to be playing in the background.

Sets of vintage china, glassware, and flatware from hotels and restaurants of yore are the main attraction, though I always keep an eye out for quirkier pieces from hospitals or ocean liners, too. Carefully chosen flea market finds, such as a French coloring book circa 1950 or a set of ceramic marbles from Italy, round out the selection. Warning: The displays here are so charming that, given a few minutes' browsing, you're likely to suddenly decide that you desperately need a vintage milk glass platter, faience café au lait bowl, or caviar server. Note that the composed, pleasant atmosphere is just a tinge louder on warm days, when the staff prop open the front door with a stack of sturdy dishware, letting in a little noise from the street.

↝ essentials

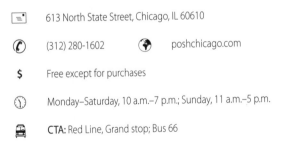

✉   613 North State Street, Chicago, IL 60610

✆   (312) 280-1602   ✪   poshchicago.com

$ Free except for purchases

🕐   Monday–Saturday, 10 a.m.–7 p.m.; Sunday, 11 a.m.–5 p.m.

🚃   **CTA:** Red Line, Grand stop; Bus 66

peaceful place 82

PRAIRIE AVENUE HISTORIC DISTRICT

Near South Side, South Side (MAP FOUR)

category ⌇ historic sites ✪ ✪

*A*s the Champs-Élysées is to Paris, Fifth Avenue is to New York City, and Rodeo Drive is to Los Angeles, so is Michigan Avenue to Chicago. But in the latter half of the 19th century, the ritziest street in the Windy City was Prairie Avenue. Wealthy residents such as railroad baron George Pullman, Philip Armour of meat-packing fame, and department store magnate Marshall Field all built mansions on a six-block stretch of it. Some of the magnificent edifices from Prairie's heyday have been lost to time, but many of them remain.

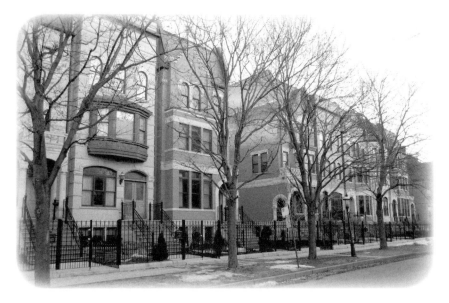

Prairie Avenue once housed the city's elite.

You can take a summertime walking tour of the neighborhood with a guide from the museum that now occupies the historic Glessner House on Prairie (see website under Essentials for dates and details), or simply stroll around by yourself. The most historic section of Prairie has been turned into a cul-de-sac, and no parking is allowed, making a walk here a quiet experience indeed. Be sure to notice the nearby Clarke House. Also available for tours, it was built in 1836 and is said to be the oldest surviving home in Chicago.

∼ essentials

▣   1800 and 1900 blocks of South Prairie Avenue, Chicago, IL 60616

☏   (312) 326-1480

⊕   webapps.cityofchicago.org/landmarksweb; glessnerhouse.org

$ Free; **combined tour of Glessner and Clarke houses:** $15

🕐   **Historic District:** Open 24/7. **Glessner House tours:** Wednesday–Sunday, 1 p.m. and 3 p.m. **Clarke House tours:** Wednesday–Sunday, noon and 2 p.m.

🚍   **CTA:** Red Line, Cermak/Chinatown stop; Bus 1, 3, or 4

peaceful place 83

PROMONTORY POINT, BURNHAM PARK

Hyde Park, South Side (MAP FOUR)

category ⌇ parks & gardens ✪ ✪

A favorite neighborhood getaway for residents of Hyde Park, what is known as The Point lies on a small peninsula extending into Lake Michigan in the vicinity of 55th Street. To find it, follow 55th Street east toward the lake, and then take the pedestrian underpass beneath Lake Shore Drive. You'll soon come to a water fountain topped by a charming statue of a fawn. Walk farther east still, and you'll come to the seawall, which is composed of large limestone blocks leading to the lake's edge.

Some hearty, warm-blooded, and adventurous sorts have been known to take advantage of the metal ladders leading down into the lake and go for an open-water

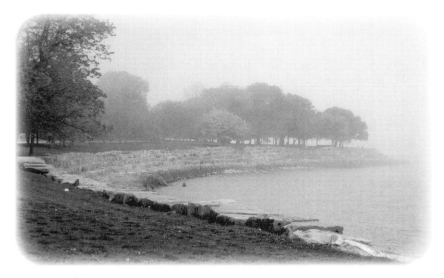

A foggy day on the lakeshore at Promontory Point

swim. However, the lack of lifeguards, as well as the presence of hidden rocks, makes a dip here a chancy prospect. Better to simply find a comfortable spot on the grass or seawall and stare out into the vast blue water. This close to the lake, the traffic noise from Lake Shore Drive is all but nonexistent. And because The Point is a peninsula, you can enjoy the novel-for-Chicago sensation of being surrounded by water on *two* sides.

essentials

▭   5491 South Lake Shore Drive, Chicago, IL 60615

🄲   (312) 747-6620

🌐   chicagoparkdistrict.com

$ Free

🕐   Daily, 6 a.m.–10:30 p.m.

🚌   **Metra Electric District:** 55th-56th-57th Street Station; **CTA:** Bus 6 or 55

peaceful place 84

RAVINIA FESTIVAL

Highland Park, Northern Suburbs (MAP FIVE)

category ↙ outdoor habitats ✪ ✪

*O*n dozens of evenings each summer, the outdoor music venue at Ravinia Park pulses with beats from beloved big-name performers such as the B-52s, Lyle Lovett, Sting, and the Indigo Girls.

But on nights when the Chicago Symphony Orchestra takes the stage, as it does several times a summer, a different mood settles over the grounds. Instead of shaking their moneymakers to "Rock Lobster" or clapping along to "Closer to Fine," festival-goers lie back on the grass or settle down in their lawn chairs and let the strains of classical music wash over them.

On these nights, it's all about peacefully soaking up the performance. In fact, that is so much the case that to minimize chatter and preserve the serene atmosphere, friendly staffers stroll around the ground holding QUIET, PLEASE signs.

Lots of Ravinia attendees like to get here early and dine on the grass before the performance starts. You can buy your dinner from one of the on-site cafés, but I much prefer bringing a simple picnic of crusty bread, sharp cheese, sweet fruit, dark chocolate, and perhaps a bottle of wine (pack a few citronella candles, too, to ward off the mosquitoes).

⌣ essentials

✉	200 Ravinia Park Road, Highland Park, IL 60035
☎	(847) 266-5100
🌐	ravinia.org (shows schedule times and performers)
$	$10–$20 (lawn seating for Chicago Symphony Orchestra)
🕐	**Chicago Symphony Orchestra:** selected evenings July–August; see website for full schedule
🚌	**Metra Union Pacific:** North Line, Ravinia Park Station

peaceful place 85

REBAR

River North, Downtown (MAP ONE)

category ↙ quiet tables ✪

*I*n the evenings, this mezzanine-level bar in the Trump Hotel grows noisy and crowded. But get here on a weekday around 4 p.m., and you'll have the refined atmosphere all to yourself. It's a lovely retreat from the outside world, especially if you're looking for a place to chat with a friend without having to shout over background noise or resort to sign language. The decor is all tasteful grays and blacks, with candles in red glass bowls on each table to liven things up a bit. But you'll likely be gazing instead at the magnificent view outside; the picture windows pan the Chicago River, producing the illusion that you're almost floating above it.

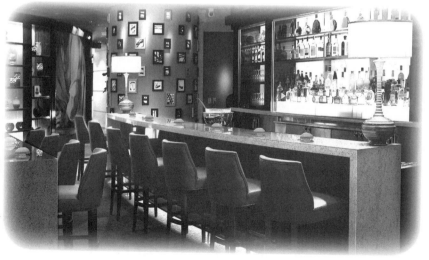

courtesy of William Huber

On weekday afternoons, Rebar offers a quiet respite.

Be forewarned that the drinks don't come cheap. A glass of the bar's signature libation, the Flor Blanco (a white sangria), runs $19, and wines by the glass range $16–$50. But what they lack in cost-effectiveness, they make up for in quality. If you prefer something nonalcoholic, the all-natural Boylen ginger ale with lime and mint is as elegant as any mojito.

essentials

✉	401 North Wabash Avenue, Chicago, IL 60611
☎	(312) 588-8000
🌐	trumpchicagohotel.com
$	**Cocktails:** $17; **beer:** $8–$12; **wine by the glass:** $16–$50
🕐	Monday–Wednesday, 4 p.m.–midnight; Thursday–Friday 4 p.m.–1 a.m.; Saturday, 3 p.m.–1 a.m.; Sunday 1 p.m.–midnight
🚌	**CTA:** Red Line, Grand stop; Bus 147

peaceful place 86

RICHARD & ANNETTE BLOCH
CANCER SURVIVORS PLAZA

The Loop, Downtown (MAP ONE)

category ↙ scenic vistas ✪ ✪

his small plaza (really more of a garden) draws visitors with its profusion of flowers, metal latticework entrance pavilions, 40-foot granite columns, and well-maintained handkerchief lawns. But to my mind, the view is the reason to visit. Stand at the plaza's northern entrance, and you are treated to the magnificent sight of the Field Museum of Natural History, lying about a mile away down Lake Shore Drive. From this distance, you can really appreciate what a monumental edifice it is. Edging the plaza's perimeters are several benches that make fine vantage points, either for taking in the Field Museum view or for just gazing at the flowers.

In addition, if you, a family member, or friend has been affected by cancer, you may appreciate the plaza's numerous plaques. They are engraved with statements meant to provide inspiration and encouragement to cancer patients and survivors, such as "Know all your options. Knowledge heals." and "Seek and accept support." To find the plaza, simply head to the intersection of Michigan Avenue and Randolph Street; then walk about 0.5 mile east on Randolph and look for the sign that announces the entrance.

↙ essentials

⌨ Upper Randolph Drive and North Harbor Drive, Chicago, IL 60601

☎ (312) 742-7648   ♞ chicagoparkdistrict.com

$ Free   ☼ Daily, 7 a.m.–11 p.m.

🚌 **Metra Electric District:** Millennium Station; **CTA:** Brown Line, Randolph/Wabash stop; Red Line, Lake stop; Bus 151

peaceful place 87

RL BAR

River North, Downtown (MAP ONE)

category ✌ quiet tables ⊗

*I*mmediately adjacent to a busy Ralph Lauren store, RL Restaurant offers upscale, old-fashioned food (lobster club sandwiches, steak accompanied by creamed spinach, and the like) in a clublike atmosphere. "It's the coziest place to eat downtown," said the friend who tipped me off, noting that he was talking about RL's bar, not its dining room proper. He was right on both counts: it would be difficult to find a more snug or more comfortable dining venue in the area.

For the most peaceful experience here, you want to follow my friend's lead and snag a seat in the quieter bar area, rather than in the restaurant itself. A fireplace warms the room in winter, and the patrons in this section seem more intent on stealing a quiet moment with their lunch and a newspaper than on noisy bantering. On cold Chicago days—and there are many—the duet of toasted cheese sandwiches, served with a hearty tomato soup, is the perfect antidote for the chill.

Unfortunately, reservations aren't taken for the bar. So unless you enjoy hovering in the lobby awaiting an empty stool, it's wisest to treat yourself to an early meal at 11 a.m.

✌ essentials

| ✉ | 115 East Chicago Avenue, Chicago, IL 60611 |

| ✆ | (312) 475-1100 | 🌐 | rlrestaurant.polo.com |

| $ | Lunch entrées: $12–$41 | 🕐 | Bar: Daily, 11 a.m.–midnight |

| 🚌 | CTA: Red Line, Chicago stop; Bus 151 |

peaceful place 88

ROBUST COFFEE LOUNGE

Woodlawn, South Side (MAP FOUR)

category ↙ quiet tables ✪

*C*an a venue with the name Robust belong in a book about peaceful places? In this
case, yes. Also, the listings in this book aside, not all of Chicago's great coffee shops
lie on the North Side, and this café in the Woodlawn neighborhood proves it.

The contemporary, laid-back vibe at Robust, which I'd sum up as community hip-
ster, draws a diverse clientele. Here, students, faculty, and staff from the nearby University of Chicago mix with neighborhood residents to enjoy an impressive array of hearty
sandwiches and other fare. However, because Robust is a little under the radar, there
seem to be fewer laptop users here than at other coffee shops in the city, meaning more

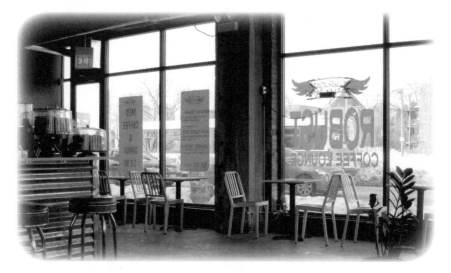

The streamlined surroundings at Robust Coffee Lounge

open tables for you. Leather chairs and a coffee table form a living room–like area that all but audibly invites you to sit down and chill out for a while. Easy parking and free Wi-Fi add to the restful atmosphere.

Just be sure to get here well before the local schools let out around 3:30, when it's not unusual for teenagers to loudly flock inside in search of snacks. And with offerings such as corned beef on rye, or peanut butter, banana, and bacon on challah, who can blame them?

↷ essentials

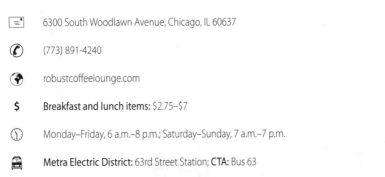

6300 South Woodlawn Avenue, Chicago, IL 60637

(773) 891-4240

robustcoffeelounge.com

$ Breakfast and lunch items: $2.75–$7

Monday–Friday, 6 a.m.–8 p.m.; Saturday–Sunday, 7 a.m.–7 p.m.

Metra Electric District: 63rd Street Station; **CTA:** Bus 63

peaceful place 89

ROCKEFELLER CHAPEL

Hyde Park, South Side (MAP FOUR)

category ⌣ spiritual enclaves ✪ ✪ ✪

*C*hapel seems far too modest a term for this Gothic edifice festooned with stone sculptures, stained glass, and scarlet-and-gold banners. Built between 1925 and 1928 thanks to a $1.5 million gift from the United States' first billionaire—oil magnate John D. Rockefeller—it can seat 1,700. The site also houses one of the world's largest

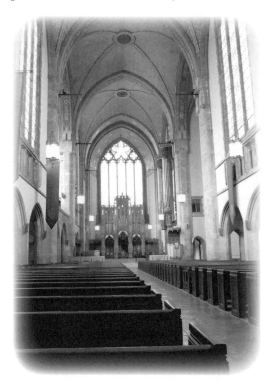

musical instruments, the 100-ton carillon (which consists of a collection of bronze bells housed in the tower).

In addition to all this splendor, the chapel offers a wonderfully tranquil sanctuary. Barring special events, Sunday services at 11 a.m., and weekday meditation services at 8 a.m., the sanctuary is generally open for contemplation.

Don't be put off by the weight of its massive wooden doors, which require nothing more than a good tug to pry open. After you slip inside, choose a seat in one of the Appalachian oak pews. On

The Gothic-majestic sanctuary within Rockefeller Chapel

sunny days, you may find yourself soaking up not only stillness but also beams of red, gold, and blue light, thanks to the enormous stained glass window in the shape of a five-petaled rose. Tip for silence seekers: You will definitely want to skip the very loud though beautiful carillon recitals, given at noon and 6 p.m. on weekdays during the academic year.

↙ essentials

▱ 5850 South Woodlawn Avenue, Chicago, IL 60637

✆ (773) 702-2100

🌐 rockefeller.uchicago.edu

$ Free

🕐 Daily, 8 a.m.–5:30 p.m.

🚌 **Metra Electric District:** 59th Street–University of Chicago Station; **CTA:** Bus 59

peaceful place 90

THE ROOKERY

The Loop, Downtown (MAP ONE)

category ⤳ historic sites ✪

*M*any local residents, let alone visitors to the city, don't recognize the name or likeness of one of the most historic and most architecturally stunning sites in Chicago. Yet this building appears on the American Institute of Architects' list of the country's 150 favorite works of architecture. Others on that list? The White House, the Empire State Building, and the Brooklyn Bridge.

The Rookery was built in 1888 to house the offices of Burnham and Root, the architects who created the World's Columbian Exposition (the 1893 fair that put Chicago on the world map). Designed by Daniel Hudson Burnham and John Wellborn Root, it features a glass-covered court, a dramatically curving twin staircase, and an entryway remodeled in 1905 by none other than Frank Lloyd Wright.

The best way to see The Rookery is on an hour-long tour led by the Chicago Architecture Foundation. CAF docents are able to take tour participants to places in The Rookery that are normally off-limits, such as Burnham and Root's own private library. True, a group tour doesn't lend itself to moments of solitude, but this building is so majestic that you and your fellow tour takers won't be able to help being struck silent at some point—perhaps at many points.

↩ essentials

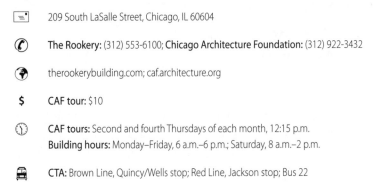

209 South LaSalle Street, Chicago, IL 60604

The Rookery: (312) 553-6100; **Chicago Architecture Foundation:** (312) 922-3432

therookerybuilding.com; caf.architecture.org

CAF tour: $10

CAF tours: Second and fourth Thursdays of each month, 12:15 p.m.
Building hours: Monday–Friday, 6 a.m.–6 p.m.; Saturday, 8 a.m.–2 p.m.

CTA: Brown Line, Quincy/Wells stop; Red Line, Jackson stop; Bus 22

peaceful place 91

ROSEHILL CEMETERY AND MAUSOLEUM

Lincoln Square, North Side (MAP TWO)

category ⌁ enchanting walks ✪ ✪ ✪

*S*ay "historic Chicago cemetery," and most people think Graceland (see page 60). But Rosehill is older and larger than its more well-known cousin, and just as architecturally beguiling. More to the purposes of this volume, it's just as peaceful as Graceland, with acre upon acre of silent landscape.

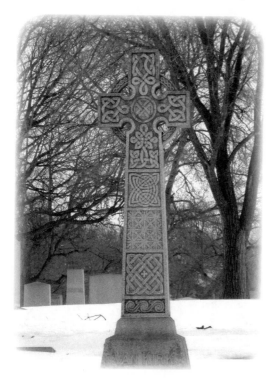

A Celtic cross marks a grave at Rosehill Cemetery.

Reach the cemetery by turning north onto Rosehill Drive from Ravenswood Avenue and entering through the arched limestone gate. You actually won't have to leave the comfort of your heated or air-conditioned vehicle, depending on the season. At 350 acres, Rosehill is so large that it is best seen from the window of a car.

Traffic on the cemetery's narrow paved roads is basically nonexistent, so you're unlikely to annoy anyone by stopping to admire an unusual gravestone—of which there are many. Numerous graves are close enough to the road that all you need to do to get a good view of them is roll down your window. Look for those marked, respectively, by a life-size metal sculpture of a deer, two stone lions, and a bench built directly into the tombstone. Or just play "spot the vintage name" game; my favorites are Braithwaite, Turnbull, and the splendid Bertram Welton Sippy, MD.

If visiting on foot, do bring a friend along. Like Graceland, Rosehill is generally safe but can feel extremely secluded.

✎ essentials

⬚ 5800 North Ravenswood Avenue, Chicago, IL 60660

☎ (773) 561-5940   ☊ rosehillcemetery.com $ Free

🕐 Monday–Saturday, 8 a.m.–5 p.m.; Sunday 9 a.m.–4 p.m.

🚌 **CTA:** Bus 22 or 50

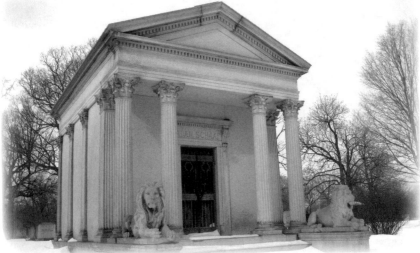

Stone lions guard a mausoleum at Rosehill Cemetery.

peaceful place 92

RUBY ROOM

Wicker Park, West Side (MAP THREE)

category ⌣ shops & services ✪ ✪ ✪

*Y*ou can't toss a bottle of conditioner in Chicago's trendy Wicker Park neighborhood without hitting a beauty salon. But how many of them also offer a Chinese herb bar, handwriting analysis, acupuncture, and astrological readings?

At the Ruby Room, clients take advantage of services such as these as well as the less exotic, more predictable offerings of haircuts, facials, and massages. I went recently for an energy healing—a 30-minute consultation with a self-declared archangel channeler. She told me that I had a yellow aura and should take baths on Wednesdays. Cynicism aside, I did actually feel lighter and more relaxed afterward. Possibly that was thanks to the hushed upscale atmosphere, which mixes oddly soothing deep-red walls with Buddha

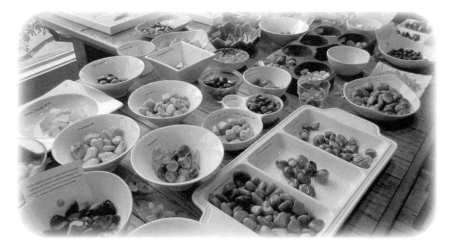

Energy crystals and gemstones for sale

statues and floor-to-ceiling cloth panels. A small retail area offers crystals, aromatherapy oils, books, and the like (alongside anti-shoplifting cards that read "Karma Is Real").

If you need more of a getaway than a 30- or 60-minute service can provide, the Ruby Room also has eight overnight guest rooms. The building houses a yoga studio as well, and guests have free access to the gym next door, making a stay here a sort of one-stop urban wellness retreat.

↵ essentials

☰⁺ 1743–45 West Division Street, Chicago, IL 60622

📞 (866) 782-9766   🌐 rubyroom.com

$ Services: $10–$175; **guest rooms:** $85–$200

🕐 Monday–Friday, 10 a.m.–9 p.m.; Saturday, 9 a.m.–7 p.m.; Sunday, 10 a.m.–7 p.m.

🚌 **CTA:** Blue Line, Division stop; Bus 50

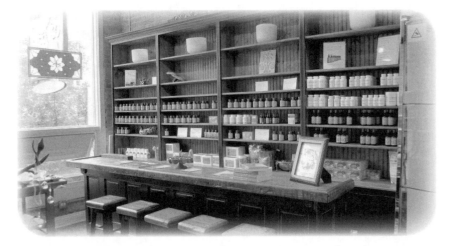

The "flower and gem essence" bar at Ruby Room

peaceful place 93

SERENE TEAZ

Elmhurst, Western Suburbs (MAP SIX)

category ✧ shops & services ✪ ✪

*T*ea connoisseurs seem spoiled for choice in Chicago's western suburbs, what with Todd & Holland Tea Merchants in Forest Park (see page 194), TeaLula in Park Ridge, and this small shop, Serene Teaz, in Elmhurst.

Located in a compact but charming shopping area near the Metra tracks, Serene Teaz features more than 100 varieties of teas and tisanes, handily organized by caffeine content. The specialty here: blends, many of them created in-house. That means that in addition to straightforward classics such as Earl Grey and oolong, you'll also find flavors such as coconut, tiramisu, apple strudel, piña colada, and (oddly enough) café latte. The Sweet

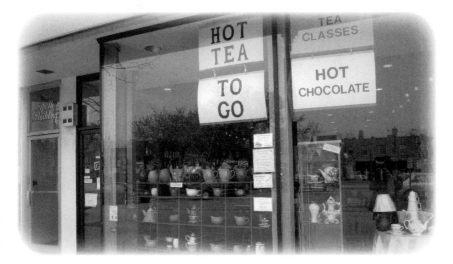

Brightly colored dishware beckons tea drinkers into Serene Teaz.

Sin tea might raise an eyebrow or bring a smile, but it's really a not-especially-naughty mix of rooibos (an herbal tea from South Africa), raspberries, rose petals, and vanilla.

Because it's possible to buy tea in quantities as small as 2 ounces here, you may find yourself loading up on lots of flavors to try (or give away). Knowledgeable staff are on hand to brew you a sample of whatever you'd like. There's a quiet café area, too, for sitting and sipping.

⌣ essentials

✉	108 West Park Avenue, Elmhurst, IL 60126
☎	(630) 833-8329
🌐	sereneteaz.com
$	$3–$15.25 per ounce
🕐	Monday–Wednesday and Friday–Saturday, 10 a.m.–5 p.m.; Thursday, 10 a.m.–8 p.m.
🚆	**Metra Union Pacific:** West Line, Elmhurst Station

peaceful place 94

SHAKESPEARE GARDEN

Evanston, Northern Suburbs (MAP FIVE)

category ⌣ parks & gardens ✪ ✪ ✪

*H*iding behind a hawthorn hedge on the campus of Northwestern University in Evanston, this meticulously tended garden exists just a few steps away from a busy sidewalk bustling with undergraduates. The first time my husband took me here, during our courtship, I couldn't believe how well its creators have secluded it, and how much a visit to it feels like stumbling into a tiny, secret, colorful world.

To find it, walk behind the university's Ford Motor Company Engineering Design Center, and look for the unassuming dirt path. Follow it east (toward Lake Michigan), and in a few moments you'll come to the garden, which is laid out in a formal square. Every last shrub and blossom here is mentioned in a Shakespearean play, such as the

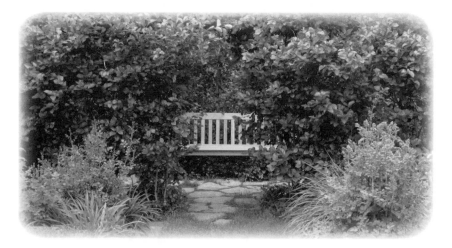

A hidden bench offers a moment of rest in the Shakespeare Garden.

fragrant rosemary ("that's for remembrance," says Ophelia in *Hamlet*). But even if you don't much care about the Swan of Avon, you'll still enjoy the stillness and beauty found here. The garden is so small that there's not a lot of strolling to be done; instead, I like to rest on the stone bench that sits at one end of it—ideally at twilight, the better to contemplate the fireflies that wink among the flowers then.

Note: This is a popular spot for proposals, so be prepared to make a tactful retreat if you see anyone holding a suspiciously small jewelry box.

⌣ essentials

🖃	Just east of Northwestern University's Ford Motor Company Engineering Design Center, 2133 Sheridan Road, Evanston, IL 60208
✆	(847) 866-7645
⊕	northwestern.edu/about/historic-moments/campus/shakespeare-garden.html
$	Free
🕐	Daily, sunrise–sunset
🚌	**CTA:** Purple Line, Noyes stop; Bus 201

peaceful place 95

SHEDD AQUARIUM

Museum Campus, Downtown (MAP ONE)

category ↝ museums & galleries ✪

Lounging sea otters, lazily throbbing jellyfish, gliding manta rays—they all invite onlookers to slip into a peacefully playful mood. But the hordes of shrieking schoolchildren that frequently pack this beautiful aquarium can make a trip here anything but serene—unless you know when to visit.

Sunday morning is by far the quietest time to enjoy the Shedd. If your schedule doesn't permit that time slot, then aim to arrive at opening time on a weekday in the fall or winter, when fewer school groups are traipsing through. For the quietest, most secluded experience, go to the underwater viewing area in the Oceanarium portion of the aquarium, where you can sit on a comfortable bench in semidarkness and watch, for as long as you like, smiling Pacific white-sided dolphins spin and slice through the water. Bonus: Cell phones don't work in this area, meaning that there are no annoying ringtones to interrupt the experience.

Another serenity-inducing stop here is the tidepool habitat, also in the Oceanarium. There's just something about watching a sea anemone's fronds waving in the (artificial) current that lowers one's blood pressure. Afterward, weather permitting, skip the frenetic food court in favor of a seat on the outside terrace of the on-site Soundings Café (open Friday–Sunday, 11 a.m.–4 p.m.). (Soundings, by the way, is named for the deep dives that whales make, not for any noises that might disturb your experience.)

⌁ essentials

☰   1200 South Lake Shore Drive, Chicago, IL 60605

☎   (312) 939-2438

🌐   sheddaquarium.org

$ **Adults and children age 12 and older:** $8–$34.95; **children ages 3–11:** $6–$25.95

🕓   **Memorial Day weekend–June 30:** Daily, 9 a.m.–6 p.m.
July 1–Labor Day weekend: Daily, 8:30 a.m.–6 p.m.
Early September–late May: Monday–Friday, 9 a.m.–5 p.m.;
Saturday–Sunday, 9 a.m.–6 p.m.

🚌   **CTA:** Bus 146

peaceful place 96

THE SHOPS AT NORTH BRIDGE GUEST LOUNGE
Magnificent Mile, Downtown (MAP ONE)

category ↲ shops & services ✪

*S*ometimes the most centrally located getaways aren't the ones in plain sight. That's the case with the guest lounge at The Shops at North Bridge, a vertical mall on the Magnificent Mile. Commonly called the Nordstrom building, thanks to its anchor store, the mall is frequently jammed with browsers seeking goods from Louis Vuitton, Benetton, and other high-end shops.

When you've been accidentally whacked by someone else's Sephora shopping bag a few too many times, head to the first-floor Nordstrom entrance and look for the array of café tables. Then do an about-face. What you want is hiding directly opposite, just behind the booths hawking jewelry and expensive moisturizers. Venture back there, and you'll find the mall's official guest lounge: a small, quiet sitting area that's surprisingly easy to overlook if you don't know about it. We're not talking a luxurious oasis here; it's simply a less noisy retreat with a few comfortable couches. But when you're all shopped out and ready to trade your purchases just for a place to sit down in peace and quiet, and perhaps enjoy examining your new treasures, it's priceless. Tranquility tip: Purchase a cup of that cappuccino to take over to your peaceful couch.

↲ essentials

▤	520 North Michigan Avenue, Chicago, IL 60611
☎	(312) 222-1622 ⊕ theshopsatnorthbridge.com $ Free
☼	Monday–Saturday, 10 a.m.–8 p.m.; Sunday, 11 a.m.–6 p.m.
☐	CTA: Red Line, Grand stop; Bus 151

peaceful place 97

THE SHRINE OF CHRIST'S PASSION

Indiana, Farther Afield (MAP SEVEN)

category ↝ spiritual enclaves ✪ ✪

*A*bout an hour's drive south of Chicago lies The Shrine of Christ's Passion, a collection of 40 life-size bronze sculptures that depict the death, resurrection, and ascension of Jesus. Arranged along a 0.5-mile trail, they are meant to inspire viewers to reflect on their faith. But the sculptures are so well crafted, and the setting so beautiful, that it's worth a stop to see them no matter what your religious persuasion (or lack thereof).

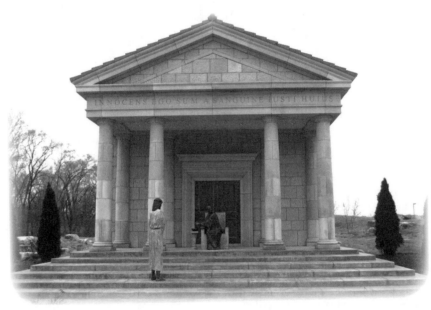

Life-size scenes from the life of Jesus are on display at the Shrine of Christ's Passion.

The trail has been landscaped so that no sculpture can be seen from any other, to permit a more solitary experience. Some of them are interactive; you can actually (and surprisingly) sit on an empty seat at a table with Jesus at *The Last Supper* piece, for example. And the sculpture titled *The First Station* permits you to walk up the steps of the temple where Pontius Pilate symbolically washed his hands after condemning Jesus to death. Visitors can contemplate each scene in silence, or press a button at a listening station to hear a devotion by Chicago news anchorman Bill Kurtis. The shrine is open year-round, and during the short days of winter, lighting illuminates the path after dark.

essentials

✉	10630 Wicker Avenue (US 41), St. John, IN 46373
☏	(219) 365-6010
🌐	shrineofchristspassion.org
$	Free
🕐	Daily, 10 a.m.–5 p.m. (until 8 p.m. on Thursdays in summer)
🚌	n/a

peaceful place 98

SKATING IN THE SKY

Magnificent Mile, Downtown (MAP ONE)

category ✂ urban surprises ✪

*I*f you love taking a twirl or two on the ice—but hate the cold and crowds—it's time to take a look up. January–March, what's reputed to be the world's highest ice rink sits on the 94th floor of the John Hancock Building. Make that "ice" rink, in quotes; what you're really skat-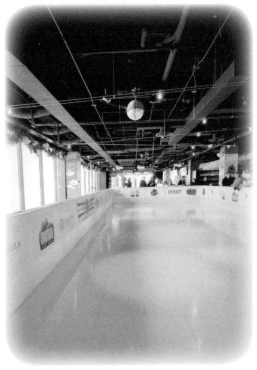ing on here is a synthetic material that doesn't melt at room temperature, meaning that you don't even have to wear a coat if you don't want to. The rink's small size doesn't allow room for showboating, so any hotshots who happen to be on the ice with you can't ruin your fun with an ill-timed triple axel. It also means that this is less a venue for serious exercise than it is simply a place to enjoy the novelty of quietly gliding on skates more than 1,000 feet above the city. Weekdays before 3 p.m. offer your best chance of having the rink either all to yourself or with

A tiny rink awaiting skaters in the John Hancock Building

only a few other skaters for company. If you work nearby, consider a short lunchtime skating session as the perfect peaceful break during a busy day.

⌣ essentials

875 North Michigan Avenue, Chicago, IL 60611

(312) 751-3681

hancockobservatory.com

25-minute skating session: $5 (must be purchased in addition to $10–$15 general observatory admission); **skate rental:** $1

January–March: Daily, 9 a.m.–11 p.m. (last admission 10:30 p.m.)

CTA: Red Line, Chicago stop; Bus 151

peaceful place 99

SKOKIE NORTHSHORE SCULPTURE PARK

Skokie, Northern Suburbs (MAP FIVE)

category ↲ enchanting walks ✪

I commuted past this park every day, twice a day, for years, without realizing it
was a park. Instead, I thought it consisted of nothing more than a series of large
sculptures, placed along McCormick Boulevard between Dempster Street and Touhy
Avenue, for the entertainment of drivers. Au contraire.

Once I stopped driving past it and started meandering through it, I understood that
this 2-mile swath is a park unto itself, complete with walking paths, bike trails, and picnic
areas. And, of course, there are the sculptures—all 65 of them, and each one different
in color, size, scope, and shape.

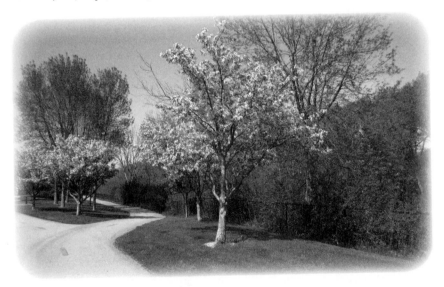

The park's paved trail leads past flowering trees.

Traffic on busy McCormick Boulevard keeps the park from ever being truly silent. Still, the other side of the park is bordered by nothing noisier than the North Shore Channel canal, and in many places the walking path veers as far from the street as space will allow.

The park consists of four 0.5-mile sections. On sunny days, it's good to keep in mind that the section between Main Street and Oakton Street is the shadiest.

↺ essentials

⌨   McCormick Boulevard between Dempster Street and Touhy Avenue, Skokie, IL 60076

☎   (847) 679-4265

🌐   sculpturepark.org

$ Free

🕒   Daily, sunrise–sunset

🚌   **CTA:** Bus 97

peaceful place 100

THE SKYDECK, WILLIS TOWER

The Loop, Downtown (MAP ONE)

category ⌣ urban surprises ✪ ✪ ✪

*H*ow does the Willis (formerly Sears) Tower, one of the most jam-packed tourist attractions in Chicago, qualify as a peaceful place? Because there's now a way to experience it in true quiet—at breakfast time.

With advance reservations, you and up to three companions can enjoy a private, catered breakfast on one of The Skydeck's four ledges, or decks. Four important points: The ledges are completely enclosed, they are made of clear glass engineered to be extra-durable, they extend 4.3 feet from the side of the tower itself, and they are located on the tower's 103rd floor—1,353 feet above Wacker Drive and the Chicago River.

Make your reservation as far in advance as possible, and be prepared to dine before The Skydeck is open to the public—that is, between 6:45

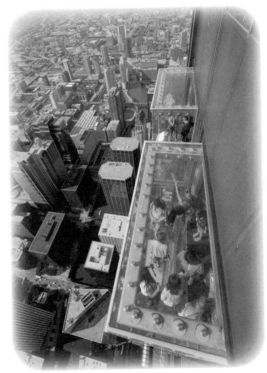

courtesy of Willis Tower

Skydeck visitors seem to float above the city.

and 8:45 a.m. (until 9:45 a.m. October–March). Though it's a pricey ($125 per person) experience, it's hands-down the quietest way to partake of the majestic view from the tower. No jostling and no waiting in line; just you, a friend or two, a lavish breakfast, and enough time to really soak in the scene far below you.

↙ essentials

⌷ 233 South Wacker Drive, Chicago, IL 60606

✆ (312) 875-9803

🌎 theskydeck.com

$ **Breakfast** (general admission included): Monday–Friday, $125 per person; Saturday–Sunday, $195 per person.
General admission: Adults and children age 12 and older: $17; children ages 3–11: $11.

🕐 Call for available times for breakfast; reservations required.
Skydeck: April–September, daily, 9 a.m.–10 p.m.;
October–March, daily, 10 a.m.-8 p.m.

🚌 **CTA:** Red Line, Jackson stop; Brown Line, Quincy stop; Bus 22

peaceful place 101

SMITH MUSEUM OF STAINED GLASS WINDOWS

Streeterville, Downtown (MAP ONE)

category ✎ museums & galleries ✪ ✪

*F*erris wheel! IMAX theater! Fun house maze! Boat cruises! With attractions such as these, plus a slew of food stands and souvenir shops, it's little wonder that few visitors to Navy Pier (Chicago's number-one tourist attraction) make it to the on-site Smith Museum of Stained Glass Windows. That's a shame, because this small, free museum features the chance to see incredible works of stained glass close up. On the other hand, it's nice to know that the few who do make it here find a rare respite from the hubbub that generally accompanies any excursion to the pier.

Said to be the only museum in the country dedicated solely to stained glass, it features both secular and religious works. Many of the former come from homes of wealthy Chicagoans built between the mid-1880s and 1915, when stained glass was fashionable in private buildings.

In the darkened Driehaus Gallery, you can see several Tiffany windows, backlit for dramatic effect, and learn how Louis Comfort Tiffany used glass not to paint *on* but to paint *with*.

Another don't-miss: an enormous window that graced the historic World's Columbian Exposition in 1893. Titled *Massachusetts Mothering the Coming Woman of Liberty, Progress, and Light*, it's a breathtaking visual representation of early American feminism. If that's not quite your speed, look instead for the modern stained glass portraits of Michael Jordan and Martin Luther King Jr. Either way, you'll have the chance to catch your breath away from the masses on the rest of Navy Pier.

essentials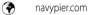

☰ 600 East Grand Avenue, Chicago, IL 60611

✆ (312) 595-5300

🌐 navypier.com

$ Free

🕐 Sunday–Thursday, 10 a.m.–8 p.m.; Friday–Saturday, 10 a.m.–10 p.m.

🚌 **CTA:** Bus 29, 65, 66, or 124 (Memorial Day–Labor Day, a free trolley runs between Navy Pier and various downtown locations; see above website for details.)

peaceful place 102

SPACE TIME TANKS
Lincoln Park, North Side (MAP TWO)
category ⌣ urban surprises ✪ ✪ ✪

*W*hen you desperately need to get away from it all, there's no more "away" place to get than a flotation tank. Don't picture a swimming pool: the tanks at Space Time are small, private, and filled with a few inches of heavily salted water. You enter a private room, disrobe, take a shower, climb into your tank, and close its door behind you.

As you lie back in the warm water, you'll be astounded by how immediately your body pops to the surface, courtesy of 800 pounds of dissolved Epsom salts. And then

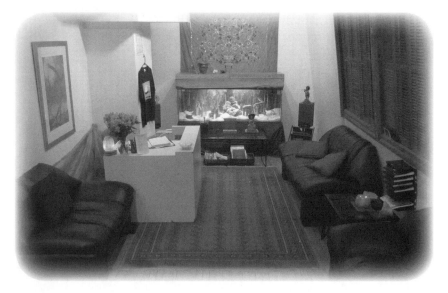

The welcoming waiting room at Space Time Tanks

what? Not a whole lot, and that's the point. You can't see anything, you can hear very little, and after a while, you even become less aware of the feeling of the water, which is heated to skin temperature for just that purpose. Some people say that floating gives them creative inspiration. Others say that it helps them remember or retain information. Still others, like me, find that it's simply a deeply relaxing way to spend an hour; I even drift off.

No worries—the water is so buoyant that it would be impossible to drown, and it's a much less claustrophobic experience than you might think: the tanks are 8 feet long, 4 feet high, and 4 feet wide, and fresh air is pumped in through vents.

One important tip: Wear the supplied earplugs, or you'll be cleaning salt crystals out of your ears afterward.

essentials

2526 North Lincoln Avenue, Chicago, IL 60614

(773) 472-2700

chicagoflotationtanks.com

$ **1-hour flotation sessions:** $50 each; packages available

Monday–Friday, noon–9 p.m.; Saturday, 10:30 a.m.–9 p.m.; Sunday, 10:30 a.m.–6 p.m.

CTA: Red Line, Fullerton stop; Bus 22

peaceful place 103

THE SPICE HOUSE
Evanston, Northern Suburbs (MAP FIVE)
category ↙ shops & services ✪ ✪

*E*ven if you bake (or, for that matter, cook) only once a year, The Spice House holds treasures for you. Ceylon cloves, Chinese anise, Jamaican allspice, Vietnamese cinnamon, and every imaginable variation of vanilla—beans, extract, paste, powder, and sugar—are just the beginning.

The Evanston location of this family business, now more than half a century old, houses shelf upon shelf of enormous glass jars, some filled with single spices and some with house-made blends. Especially fun among the latter: the Brisket of Love BBQ Seasoning Rub, created by one staff member for his fiancée, and the Chicago Deep Dish Pizza Pizzazz blend, meant to re-create the flavor of your favorite slice.

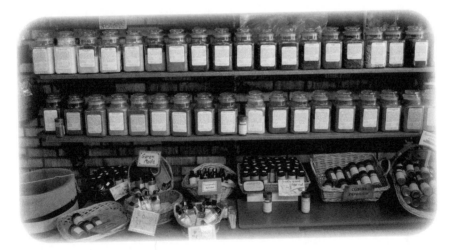

From fennel to fenugreek, The Spice House has a flavor for everything.

But what makes this a rich, peaceful sensory experience rather than just a shopping excursion? The hushed atmosphere, for one; the pervasive scent of spices, for another; the free samples of candied ginger, crystallized honey, and roasted cacao nibs, for yet another. The Spice House also has locations in Chicago; Milwaukee, Wisconsin; and Geneva, Illinois, but the Evanston branch wins my vote for most atmospheric.

essentials

☰ 1941 Central Street, Evanston, IL 60201

☎ (847) 328-3711

🌐 thespicehouse.com

$ Free except for purchases

🕐 Monday–Friday, 9 a.m.–6:30 p.m.; Saturday, 10 a.m.–5 p.m.; Sunday, 11 a.m.–3 p.m.

🚌 **CTA:** Purple Line, Central stop; Bus 201

peaceful place 104

ST. ANDREW CHAPEL

River North, Downtown (MAP ONE)

category ↶ spiritual enclaves ✪ ✪ ✪

*T*ucked on the north exterior of the grand St. James' Cathedral sit two heavy red doors. They guard what may well be the quietest space in this noisy neighborhood—the wee St. Andrew Chapel, a far more intimate and restful place than the cathedral above it. The moment those doors shut behind you, nearly all street racket vanishes as you step down into the small, still space. Its stone arches, stained glass windows, carved prayer rail, and embroidered kneeler cushions will make you feel a bit as if you've wandered into some silent corner of a medieval abbey, and no wonder: that's just what the chapel was modeled after when it was built in 1913. The altar, elaborately painted with scenes from the life of St. Andrew, only adds to the atmosphere.

The dark wooden pews seat all of 40 people, but you'll likely have the place to yourself for a bit of meditation or just a quiet moment (unless you've stepped in during one of the six weekly worship services—check the information board inside for days and times).

↶ essentials

🖃	65 East Huron Street, Chicago, IL 60611
✆	(312) 787-7360
🌐	www.saintjamescathedral.org
$	Free
🕐	Daily, 9 a.m.–4 p.m.
🚌	**CTA:** Red Line, Chicago stop; Bus 151

peaceful place 105

STARVED ROCK STATE PARK

North-central Illinois, Farther Afield (MAP SEVEN)

category ⌇ day trips & overnights ✪ ✪

*T*hough this state park lies a little more than 2 hours' drive southwest of the city, a surprising number of Chicagoans adore it. Perhaps because it's just far away enough to make you feel as if you've really left the city, without being so far away that

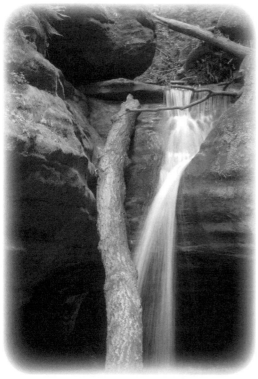

courtesy of Kathy Casstevens

the trip turns into a logistical drag. Or perhaps because the park is home to a population of beautiful bald eagles, lovely waterfalls, and vivid wildflowers. Or perhaps because you can enjoy the solitude of a long hike to one of the park's many canyons during the day, and then retire at night to the creature comforts of the lodge, which features an indoor pool and hot tub.

A nice advantage, especially in the Midwestern climate: This park is as stunning in winter as it is in summer (not to mention much less crowded). During the coldest months, you may be lucky

One of many waterfalls within Starved Rock State Park

enough to encounter water hanging in beautiful ice formations off canyon walls. Cold weather is also the best time to spy the bald eagles, which are generally seen hunting near the butte that gives the park its name, Starved Rock. (Various legends are ascribed to its name, but none is very well authenticated.)

essentials

2668 East 875th Road, Oglesby, IL 61348

(800) 868-7625

starvedrockstatepark.org

Free; lodging begins at $70 per night

Day use: Daily, 7 a.m.–9 p.m. **Trails:** Daily, sunrise–sunset

n/a

peaceful place 106

ST. PETER'S IN THE LOOP
The Loop, Downtown (MAP ONE)
category ↝ spiritual enclaves ✪ ✪ ✪

*U*nlike many other places of worship, the sanctuary of this Catholic parish is filled with activity even on weekdays. But the atmosphere here is so serenely sacred that even the frequent coming and going of people can't mar it. Some come to make confession, others to light a candle, and others to say a silent prayer, but no one will mind if your only goal is to sit quietly in a pew and absorb the hushed mood. (Tip: Be careful with any belongings in this large, silent space, as a dropped pen sounds like a gunshot.) Certainly there's enough to look at, between the paintings of the stations of the cross, the statues of Jesus and Mary, and the shrines to the religious figures known as the Little Flower and the Infant of Prague. Then, too, you may see Franciscan friars walking about in their brown robes or black-clad priests kneeling in the pews as they pray the rosary. Masses are said seven times daily on weekdays, twice on Saturdays, and four times on Sundays. Visit between Masses if quiet time is all you're after.

↝ essentials

📧 110 West Madison Street, Chicago, IL 60602

✆ (312) 372-5111

🌐 stpetersloop.org

$ Free

🕐 Monday–Friday, 5:30 a.m.–7 p.m.; Saturday, 11 a.m.–7 p.m.; Sunday, 8:30 a.m.–7 p.m.; see website for worship service times

🚆 **CTA:** Blue Line, Washington stop; Bus 22

peaceful place 107

ST. THERESE CHINESE CATHOLIC MISSION
Chinatown, South Side (MAP FOUR)
category ⌣ spiritual enclaves ✪ ✪ ✪

*W*hether for personal reflection or just to admire its beauty, visitors are welcome to sit quietly in the sanctuary of this small, unusual Chinatown parish. However, because the doors are generally locked, you are advised to call ahead and make sure that

a staff member will be available to let you in. The beauty you'll find inside is well worth that small effort.

The church began life in 1904 as Santa Maria Incoronata, a parish for Italian immigrants, as the names on the stained glass windows (Rosario, Urso, and Morelli) attest. However, the neighborhood steadily turned from Italian to Chinese in the years following World War II. By 1963, Santa Maria Incoronata had become the St. Therese Chinese Mission.

The modern sanctuary blends those historic influences charmingly. On special

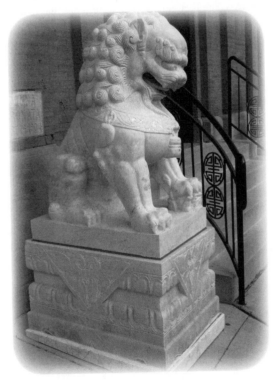

A stylized lion guards the entrance to the St. Therese Chinese Catholic Mission in Chinatown.

occasions, red cloth panels embroidered with gold Chinese characters flank the chancel (altar area). If you look up at the arches on either side of the pews, you'll see more Chinese characters painted within otherwise traditional Italian designs. In front of some of the statues of saints, you may spot blue-and-white porcelain vases of Asian design holding offerings of flowers. And outside, two Chinese lion statues guard the entrance.

essentials

218 West Alexander Street, Chicago, IL 60616

(312) 842-6777

sttheresechinatown.org

$ Free

Call to arrange visit. **English-language Masses:** Daily, 8 a.m.; Saturday, 5 p.m.; Sunday, 8 a.m. and 9:30 a.m.; see website for schedule of Masses in other languages.

CTA: Red Line, Cermak/Chinatown stop; Bus 62

peaceful place 108

SULZER REGIONAL LIBRARY

Lincoln Square, North Side (MAP TWO)

category ↝ reading rooms ✪ ✪ ✪

*D*on't be fooled by the bustling atmosphere on the first floor; this charming and well-stocked neighborhood library sports several pockets of quiet.

After entering, skirt the circulation desk and its chatter and ascend the blue staircase, pausing on the landing, if you like, to smile at the mildly cross-eyed bust of Abraham Lincoln displayed there. Once upstairs, head to your right, through the reference section, to the east-facing bank of windows. While only a few tables stand here, it's more hushed and more secluded than the periodicals section (the other main reading area), and the view of the quiet, tree-lined street outside is a lovely one.

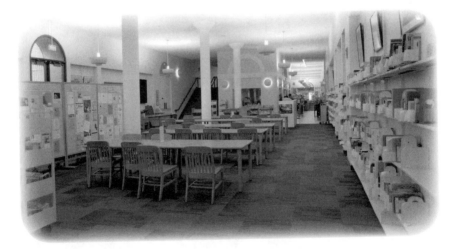

The first-floor reading area at Sulzer Regional Library

If you're really looking to cordon yourself off, take the elevator up another story to the small indoor deck that houses the local history collection. (Note: The local history collection is only open Tuesday, 2–5 p.m., and by appointment.) Hardly anyone seems to take advantage of the several reading chairs here, some of which are painted with traditional Swedish designs that reflect the neighborhood's cultural origins. From your vantage point up here, the rest of the world will seem pleasantly far removed.

↙ essentials

🖃	4455 North Lincoln Avenue, Chicago, IL 60625
✆	(312) 744-7616
🌐	chipublib.org
$	Free
🕐	Monday–Thursday, 9 a.m.–9 p.m.; Friday–Saturday, 9 a.m.–5 p.m.; Sunday, 1–5 p.m.
🚌	**CTA:** Brown Line, Western stop; Bus 11

peaceful place 109

TADAO ANDO GALLERY, THE ART INSTITUTE OF CHICAGO

The Loop, Downtown (MAP ONE)

category ↶ museums & galleries ✪ ✪ ✪

*E*nter this small, dimly lit gallery within The Art Institute's Asian section, and you'll find yourself making your way through a square formed by 16 floor-to-ceiling pillars of dark wood. They're meant to evoke the entryway to a traditional Japanese home, but to me, at least, they produce the impression that I'm slipping through a grove of trees. Either way, they force one to slow down a bit, rather than rushing in and out of the gallery with barely a glance at its contents. That's a good thing, because this is one of the loveliest and most secluded environments within the often noisy, crowded Art Institute. The gallery houses a rotating selection of truly beautiful Japanese ceramics, both ancient and modern, that deserve attention.

One of the pieces you may see: Hideaki Miyamura's *Bottle with Gold Glaze*, which immediately draws the eye with its luminescence. A curved wooden bench provides a comfortable seat from which to contemplate this and other pieces that take a little longer to absorb. Afterward, if you're in the mood to seek out a similarly peaceful spot, try heading downstairs to the photography section, which is often much quieter than the larger upstairs galleries.

⌣ essentials

▤   111 South Michigan Avenue, Chicago, IL 60603

𝒞   (312) 443-3600

🌍   artic.edu

$ **Adults:** $18; **seniors age 65 and older, students, and children age 14 and older:** $12; **children age 13 and younger:** free; **first and second Wednesday of every month:** free

🕐   Monday–Wednesday and Friday–Sunday, 10:30 a.m.–5 p.m.; Thursday, 10:30 a.m.–8 p.m.

🚌   **Metra Electric District:** Van Buren Street Station; **CTA:** Brown, Green, Orange, Pink, or Purple lines, Adams/Wabash stop; Bus 151

peaceful place 110

THOUSAND WAVES SPA FOR WOMEN

Lake View, North Side (MAP TWO)

category ↙ shops & services ✪ ✪ ✪

*I*t's the aroma of this day spa that starts relaxing me the minute I walk through the door. Wafting toward me is Thousand Waves's faint but soothing blend of eucalyptus (from the steam room) and lavender (from the herbal wraps).

Massages and herbal wraps are available, but if you're watching your wallet, you can just come for a spa bath visit, which includes 3 hours of access to the hot tub, sauna, steam room, and relaxation room. That last is a large, quiet space with comfy chairs, soft

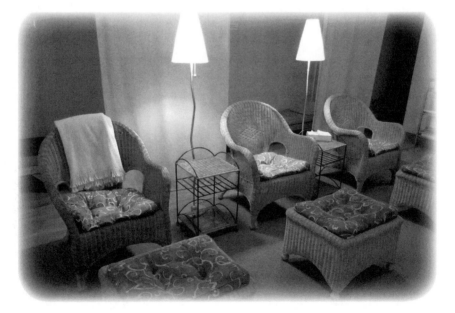

The relaxation room at Thousand Waves Spa

blankets, private cubbies with cots for napping, herbal tea, and magazines. For the ultimate relaxation experience, sit in the steam room for as long as you can stand it—in my case, that's all of 3 minutes—then exit, plunge yourself into a brief freezing-cold shower, and towel off. You'll sleep like a baby that night, I promise.

Be forewarned that this women-only spa is a clothing-optional environment. Bathing suits are allowed, and the staff supply cotton kimono-style robes to walk around in, but in the hot tub, sauna, steam room, and locker room, you'll almost certainly encounter one or more ladies in the buff.

↵ essentials

⌨ 1212 West Belmont Avenue, Chicago, IL 60657

📞 (773) 549-0700

🌐 thousandwavesspa.com

$ Spa treatments: $60–$135; spa baths: $20

🕐 Tuesday, noon–5:30 p.m.; Wednesday–Thursday, noon–9 p.m.;
Friday–Sunday, 10 a.m.–7 p.m.

🚌 CTA: Red Line, Belmont stop; Bus 77

peaceful place 111

TODD & HOLLAND TEA MERCHANTS
Forest Park, Western Suburbs (MAP SIX)
category ◡⁖ shops & services ⊙ ⊙

*W*hether you prefer oolong or jasmine, green gunpowder or plain old Earl Grey, Todd & Holland has a tea for you. On well-organized shelves stand jars of some 200 loose-leaf varieties, some single-source, some blended. Two teas are always brewed and ready for sampling too. The knowledgeable staff are happy to make suggestions based on your preferences. I recently confessed my sweet tooth to them and came away with one black tea redolent of amaretti cookies, another that tastes of chocolate, and a green tea flavored with cherry pieces—delightful.

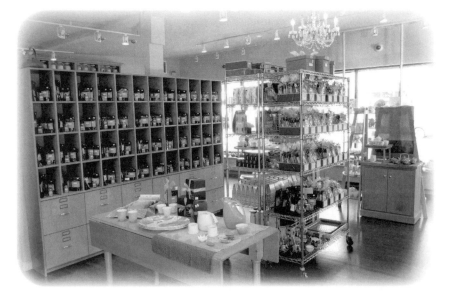

Loose-leaf teas are carefully categorized at Todd & Holland.

But when you find your favorite, act fast: as an employee told me, "next year it may not taste the same" because tea's flavor, like that of wine, is influenced by the weather of the place it's grown. Also available in the bright, cheerful store are beautiful teapots and teacups, a few specialty foods (such as locally made jams), and sundry gift items such as tea samplers. There's something about tea that tends to send people into a contemplative state or, at least, that's what you might conclude after experiencing the pleasantly hushed atmosphere here.

⌣ essentials

▤ 7311 West Madison Street, Forest Park, IL 60130

🕐 (800) 747-8327

🌐 todd-holland.com

$ **Most teas:** $22–$50 per 4 ounces

🕐 Monday–Wednesday and Friday, 10 a.m.–6 p.m.; Thursday, 10 a.m.–8 p.m.; Saturday, 10 a.m.–5 p.m.

🚆 **Metra Union Pacific:** West Line, Oak Park Station; **CTA:** Blue Line, Harlem/Forest Park stop

peaceful place 112

UIC SKYSPACE

University Village, West Side (MAP THREE)

category ⌣ urban surprises ★

To find one of the most intriguing sights on Chicago's West Side, head to the busy intersection of Roosevelt Road and Halsted Street. On its southwest corner, you'll discover the University of Illinois at Chicago's Earl L. Neal Plaza, and you can't miss the towering, red, elliptical structure in the middle of it.

That formation is a skyspace—an outdoor chamber supported by columns and containing a large egg-shaped hole in its ceiling. Artist James Turrell has created more than

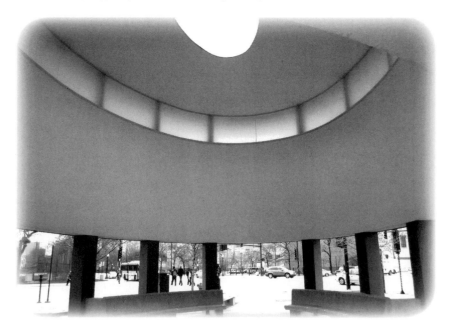

Interior of the UIC Skyspace

20 of them, and this is one of only two in the Midwest (the other is in Minnesota). A unique feature is its accessibility year-round from the public street.

As you'll discover when you step inside this one, a skyspace frames a slice of the heavens in such a way that they appear to be a constantly changing painting. Even on an overcast day, if you look long enough, you'll see differences in light, color, and patterns. You will enjoy a particularly rewarding sight at sunrise and sunset, and for the quietest ambience, I recommend the former. Concrete benches beneath the skyspace offer a place to relax during your heavenward contemplations.

✌ essentials

▤ Corner of Halsted Street and Roosevelt Road, Chicago, IL 60608

☎ n/a

🌐 uic.edu

$ Free

🕓 Open 24/7

🚌 **Metra Burlington Northern Santa Fe (BNSF) Railway:** Halsted Station;
CTA: Blue Line, UIC-Halsted stop; Bus 8, 12, or 18

peaceful place 113

UNCOMMON GROUND
Wrigleyville, North Side (MAP TWO)
category ↙ quiet tables ✪ ✪

*T*he mostly local and organic menu here is delicious whenever you visit, whether that's during the busy dinner hour or the bustling weekend brunch. But for the quietest experience, stop by for a meal or snack during a weekday afternoon, when the only other patrons are people calmly tapping away on their laptops.

In this lively Wrigleyville neighborhood, that's no insignificant find. In winter, curl up in a leather chair by the front room's cozy fireplace; in summer, enjoy the back room and its distance from the street. Also in summer, look out front for the plants that supply the restaurant with tomatoes; it's harder to get produce that's more local than that. The absolutely do-not-miss items on the menu include the macaroni and cheese, made with *butterkase*, white Cheddar, and Swiss; the sweet-potato fries, studded with salt crystals and served with goat-cheese fondue; and the peanut-butter-mocha coffee, made with organic espresso, chocolate, steamed milk, and miniature peanut butter cups.

Before you leave, be sure to check out the unisex bathroom. It's not that you had too much caffeine: this space really is painted to look like a peaceful autumn scene, complete with three-dimensional "trees" and sculpted leaves hanging from the ceiling.

↙ essentials

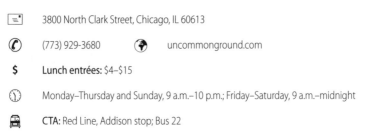

▤   3800 North Clark Street, Chicago, IL 60613

☎   (773) 929-3680   🌐   uncommonground.com

$ **Lunch entrées:** $4–$15

🕐   Monday–Thursday and Sunday, 9 a.m.–10 p.m.; Friday–Saturday, 9 a.m.–midnight

🚌   **CTA:** Red Line, Addison stop; Bus 22

peaceful place 114

UNITY TEMPLE

Oak Park, Western Suburbs (MAP SIX)

category ⌣ spiritual enclaves ✪ ✪ ✪

*D*esigned by Frank Lloyd Wright, Unity Temple arguably looks like no other house of worship you've ever seen. From outside, it resembles nothing so much as a concrete cube, albeit a strangely graceful one, adorned by columns. Wright placed the main entrance on the side of the building so that the front wall would block noise from outside—and it worked; the temple's interior is restful and quiet despite the fact that it sits on one of the busiest streets in Oak Park.

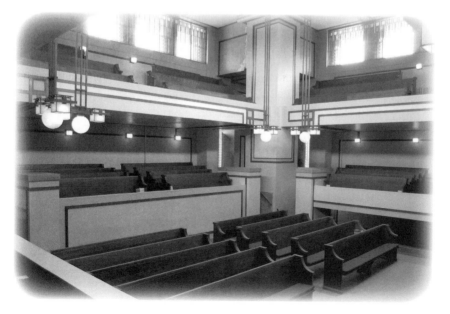

The sanctuary of Oak Park's Unity Temple

To see it, you'll have to either attend a Sunday service or take a self-guided tour for a small fee. I recommend the latter if your chief goal is to experience the temple in the most peaceful way, with as few other people around as possible. The beauty of exploring on your own is that you can sit as long as you like and take all the photos you like.

Either way, the more time you spend in the sanctuary, the more you'll appreciate Wright's attention to every detail. Round light fixtures break up the room's otherwise straight lines, while the pale yellow, pale green, and dark brown colors that Wright used evoke the serenity of nature.

Cleverly, the sanctuary is designed so that no seat is more than 40 feet from the podium, and so that latecomers to worship services can slip into the balconies without disturbing others.

essentials

✉	875 Lake Street, Oak Park, IL 60301
☎	(708) 383-8873
🌐	unitytemple.org
$	**Self-guided tours:** $9 (all of which goes to the much-needed restoration program)
🕐	**Self-guided tours:** Monday–Friday, 10:30 a.m.–4:30 p.m.; Saturday, 10 a.m.–2 p.m.; Sunday, 1–4 p.m. **Sunday worship services:** 9 a.m. and 10:45 a.m.
🚌	**CTA:** Green Line, Oak Park stop; **Metra Union Pacific:** West Line, Oak Park Station

peaceful place 115

URHAUSEN GREENHOUSES
Lincolnwood, Northern Suburbs (MAP FIVE)
category ↝ shops & services ✪ ✪

*I*n spring and summer, this 2-acre greenhouse becomes an Eden, just as it has every year since 1922, when the Urhausen family business began. Flowering plants both hang over and border the edges of seemingly endless aisles. Begonias, geraniums, verbena, petunias, impatiens, marigolds, daylilies, zinnias, snapdragons, and many other vigorously blossoming plants are for sale in baskets, flats, and pots, along with herbs and vegetable plants—all of them grown right here, not trucked in from elsewhere.

In other seasons, you won't enjoy quite such a magnificent flowering, but the conservatory atmosphere of peaceful abundance remains. Don't expect to find an array of flower-themed aprons, journals, earrings, or other trifles for sale as you might at other nurseries, however. This gardening business is all gardening business.

The greenhouse stands a bit off the beaten path in a largely residential neighborhood, and the staff (while helpful) are far from effusive. That makes it easy to pretend that you're in a secret garden alone, except for the shy gray-and-white cat who sometimes peeks at customers from behind the checkout counter. Bring your cash or checkbook, as no credit or debit cards are accepted, and pause on your way out to admire the enormous adjacent garden.

↝ essentials

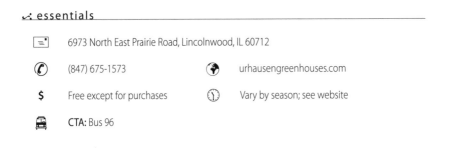

⌨ 6973 North East Prairie Road, Lincolnwood, IL 60712

☏ (847) 675-1573   🌐 urhausengreenhouses.com

$ Free except for purchases   🕐 Vary by season; see website

🚌 CTA: Bus 96

peaceful place 116

VICTORY'S BANNER
Roscoe Village, North Side (MAP TWO)
category ∿ quiet tables ⭐

*H*ow do you make a restaurant as peaceful as possible? Well, you can go upscale, with thick carpets, a minimal number of tables, and waiters trained to speak in hushed tones. Or you can have your restaurant run by students of meditation.

Seriously, this Roscoe Village vegetarian breakfast-and-lunch eatery is owned and operated by devotees of Indian spiritual teacher Sri Chinmoy, giving it what the popular local restaurant show *Check, Please!* calls a "Zen-like environment."

There seems little that is restrained, however, about the menu. It features mostly typical American fare such as omelets, French toast, chocolate-chip pancakes, and the like. Things get a little more exotic at lunch, with marinated tofu-veggie wraps and vegetarian "meat" loaf. Expect diner-style decor and cheerful servers in saris.

Meditation students or not, this place gets packed and chatty on weekends, especially during Sunday brunch, so if it's quiet you're after, aim for a weekday. Note that the restaurant closes for 10–12 days in April and again in August so the staff can go on spiritual retreats.

∿ essentials

🖃	2100 West Roscoe Street, Chicago, IL 60618
✆	(773) 665-0227 🌐 victorysbanner.com
$	Entrées: $4.95–$9.85
🕐	Monday and Wednesday–Sunday, 8 a.m.–3 p.m.
🚌	**CTA:** Brown Line, Paulina or Addison stop; Bus 50

peaceful place 117

WARNER PARK AND GARDENS

Lake View, North Side (MAP TWO)

category ∿ parks & gardens ✪ ✪

*I*gnore the feeling that you've actually strayed into someone's private yard. This small community-maintained park really is meant to be enjoyed by the general public, despite its location on a residential street between two single-family homes.

Here, a brick path surrounded by trees and flowers leads to a small gazebo, where you are welcome to sit. Or choose one of the benches scattered throughout the park. Either way, the scenery and surroundings are yours to enjoy. As a sign posted in the park reads: "Don't forget to smell the flowers and listen to the birds."

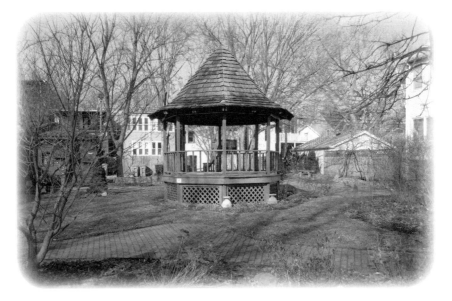

Warner Park and Gardens centers on a lovely gazebo.

Look in particular for the 100-year-old ginkgo tree (the one with the fan-shaped leaves). The community group that looks after this park does a wonderful job of keeping it well tended, making it a true breath of fresh air in the busy city. It's an especially impressive accomplishment considering how close the park lies to busy Clark Street. (Don't worry—the noise of the traffic from Clark doesn't carry as far as the park.)

⌣ essentials

▦	1446 West Warner Avenue, Chicago, IL 60613
☎	n/a
⊕	gracelandwest.org/Warner.htm
$	Free
⏱	Daily, sunrise–9 p.m.
🚌	**CTA:** Brown Line, Montrose stop; Bus 22

peaceful place 118

WAUKEGAN YACHT CLUB

Waukegan, Northern Suburbs (MAP FIVE)

category ↶ quiet tables ⭐

*U*nder most circumstances, the Waukegan Yacht Club is an exclusive establishment, open only to members. But during the lunch hour on Tuesdays–Fridays, nonmembers are welcome to the club's dining room—with its lovely setting on Waukegan Harbor. I recently took advantage of this fact and enjoyed a low-key lunch with excellent service and stellar views, all for less than what I'd usually pay for the equivalent at a downtown-Chicago restaurant.

Oddly enough, the dining room is especially enjoyable on a foggy day. That's when the mist blows romantically across the harbor, and the sight of a white sailboat ethereally skimming along the water seems like something out of a nautical fairy tale. For the quietest experience in the dining room, aim for a late lunch, at 1 p.m. or after. By then most of the diners have departed, and you

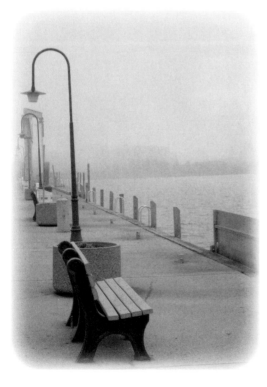

The Waukegan Yacht Club's exterior walkway along Lake Michigan

can enjoy the scenery and food (the latter mostly of the soup-and-sandwich genre) in relative solitude. After lunch, take a stroll outside by the harbor, where Canada geese and their endearingly clumsy babies toddle around the grass.

⌣ essentials

⊟   199 North Harbor Place, Waukegan, IL 60085

Ⓒ   (847) 623-4188

⊕   wyclub.com

$ **Lunch entrées:** $8.95–$15.95

🕐   Tuesday–Friday, 11:30 a.m.–2 p.m.

🚌   **Metra Union Pacific:** North Line, Waukegan Station

peaceful place 119

THE WINTER GARDEN, HAROLD WASHINGTON LIBRARY CENTER

The Loop, Downtown (MAP ONE)

category ↙ reading rooms ✪ ✪ ✪

*W*hich area of Chicago's main library you visit depends on the degree of quiet you're after. If you don't mind a fair amount of activity, the third floor (where the circulation desk and public computers are located) will do just fine. If a little bit of background noise would suit you better, head to floors four through eight.

But if only complete silence will do, you want The Winter Garden on the ninth floor. Both more stately and more bare than its name suggests, it's really a single, very large room with a lovely marble floor, and topped by a 52-foot glass dome and decorated with trees in planters. (The garden is frequently rented out for wedding receptions of up to 400 guests, if that gives you a sense of its scale.)

You'll find no books up here—just a few tables and chairs where you can work, write, read, or whatever, in near-total quiet. The glow of the sunlight coming through the glass dome is much appreciated in winter months, and there's free Wi-Fi access as well.

↙ essentials

[=] 400 South State Street, Chicago, IL 60605

✆ (312) 747-4300   ✈ chipublib.org $ Free

☾ Monday–Thursday, 9 a.m.–9 p.m.; Friday–Saturday, 9 a.m.–5 p.m.; Sunday, 1–5 p.m.

🚌 **CTA:** Brown, Purple, Orange, or Pink lines, Library stop; Bus 29

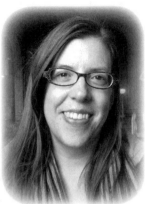

A Chicago-area resident since 1996, Anne Ford has written about travel, religion, food, and other topics for *AAA Living, Insight Guides: Chicago,* the *Chicago Tribune, Lake, Parenting, Natural Solutions, Creative Living,* AOL Travel, *Crain's Chicago Business,* and the *Chicago Reader,* among other publications. During her days as a travel editor for Rand McNally, she contributed many features to the company's iconic line of road atlases.

Ford received her master's degree in religion from the University of Chicago.